AWAKENINGS IN REAL LIFE

AWAKENINGS
in real life

Family stories of inspiration, meaning, and hope

a memoir by DAN COHEN

CURRENT WORDS PUBLISHING | LOS ANGELES

Awakenings in Real Life

Editor: Dianne Pearce
Cover art and interior design: David Yurkovich

ISBN: 978-1-957224-99-2 (paperback)
ISBN: 978-1-957224-62-6 (ePub)

Library of Congress Control Number: 2025950995

Published by Current Words Publishing, LLC
Los Angeles, California
currentwords.com

For Dad. I love you to pieces.

Table of Contents

PART 4

AWAKENINGS IN REAL LIFE

Preface

What Is an Awakening?

When you hear the term "awakening," what comes to mind? I surmise that most people think of something *big*, like a religious or spiritual awakening. And something *big* did indeed happen to my family. My dad, who was in the late stages of dementia, had a brief awakening from his condition and was very close to being his "normal self." This book will share that experience and the message of hope I believe it will give to families and caregivers of family members who suffer from Alzheimer's and dementia to know that our loved ones still *appreciate and live life*. I wrote an article about our experience, and I have received many positive, heartwarming comments, including the following:

Thank you for sharing such a heartfelt and insightful article. Your story deeply resonated with me, especially the emotional journey of caring for a loved one with dementia. The temporary awakening of your father provides a unique perspective on how moments of clarity, though fleeting, can bring immense value to both the person experiencing them and their family. I believe your reflection on how those moments, even if brief, can offer new insights into life and appreciation for what remains is powerful. It's a reminder that while we may not be able to control the progression of such diseases, we can cherish every meaningful interaction and never lose hope.

As I read your wonderful story that encapsulates so many emotions for adult children who are caregivers of parents with dementia/Alzheimer's, or for any dementia-related cognitive disorder, I praise you and your family for your bravery and dedication. I am the primary caregiver for my mom (eight years into the journey), and it is a battle to say the least. Because there are so many unknowns in this battle and on the journey, an Awakening can be a tender relief from the agonizing experiences from the stages . . . Thank you!

Wow, Dan, what a touching story. I empathize with your situation—I've been taking care of my mom since 2016, when she was diagnosed with Alzheimer's—it's such an emotional roller coaster to see our parents in this state . . . Thank you for sharing your father's story.

Thank you for writing this, and for loving your dad and continuing to include him in life . . . It takes enormous patience, presence, and love to continue to attend and give space for the positive changes to occur. This is a beautiful story, thank you again for sharing it.

So beautiful, in a bittersweet way. Your father's experience teaches us that a cure is possible and that his pre-dementia self truly is alive and well, but somehow lost in his brain.

My dad passed away in April 2016. I knew that someday I wanted to share the story and more about my dad's life with a broader audience by writing a book. I also had other experiences with Dad and his dementia where I learned many things along the way that I wanted to include in the book and share with others. However, these stories alone were not enough to fit the pages of an entire book. I sat on the idea for a number of years.

It's been ten years since I wrote the article. The article gets more views today than it did when I first wrote it. It clearly resonates with an audience. The thought of writing a book kept gnawing at me. I started to research what the term awakening means:

Merriam-Webster defines awakening as:

1: a rousing from sleep
2a: a rousing from inactivity or indifference
2b: a revival of interest in something (such as religion)
3: a coming into awareness

In a sense, my father *woke up* from his dementia, and this experience would broadly fit into definition number 1 or 2a. Dictionary.com expands on definition 3, when it states Awakening is ". . .a recognition, realization or coming into awareness of something."

Suddenly, it hit me. My father's awakening triggered an awakening *in me*. All Awakenings do not have to be *big*, but they should be inspiring, hopeful, or significant. To me, the word awakening implies a deeper meaning, beyond a rousing experience or realization. When I think of awakenings, those thoughts involve stories of enlightenment, lessons learned, deep understandings, and personal growth. So, when I used the catalyst of my dad's awakening to take a deep dive into my family's history, it involved all those things, and I wanted to share them in this book. I'm hoping that you might recognize some similar awakenings in yourself or your family, be entertained by the stories, learn from our experiences, or find meaning in your own life.

Though in many ways these are really life lessons, I think of them as mini-awakenings. I also think of them as more gifts from my dad, because without his awakening, I may never have realized all the others that had already happened in my life. All of these events, when looked at through the lens of my father's awakening, inspire me to be reflective in my own life and realize how many blessings life brings to us that we are too asleep to see. May the awakenings in your life wake you up to your blessings, as my dad's awakening woke me up to mine.

PART 1
Dad's Dementia Journey and Awakening

Prologue

When My Father Woke Up, He Woke Me Up Too

For my family, the 1990 drama *Awakenings* is not just a movie. Based on the true story of Dr. Oliver Sacks, Penny Marshall's film centers on Dr. Malcolm Sayer (played by Robin Williams) and his patient Leonard Lowe (played by Robert De Niro). In the film, Sayer uses a drug designed to treat Parkinson's Disease to awaken catatonic patients living in a Bronx hospital. The most dramatic and amazing results are found in Leonard. Although Leonard completely awakens, the results are temporary, and he reverts to his catatonic state. Dr. Sayer tells a group of hospital grant donors that although Leonard's awakening did not last, another type of awakening, "learning to appreciate and live life," had taken place, and that this is the message they should take from the event.

While not as dramatic as in the movie, my dad, who suffered from severe dementia, also had a period where he awakened. This book is about the time my dad woke up from his dementia and came back to us, and why we think it happened. But most of all, this book is about the profound impact Dad's awakening had, and still has, on me and my family. When my dad woke up, it was a gift I thought was beyond reach, and the greatest gift I have ever received, beyond having my dad as my dad, and having all of the wonderful people in my family. There isn't a formula here: *How you can wake up your loved one from dementia in three easy steps*, but there is a suggestion on what you can do, in your life, and in the lives of those you love, to be sure you are all awake, and never miss any of the many awakenings life brings to all of us, so many times over; little miraculous gifts that we are too worried, or distracted, or busy to notice. It puts me in mind of the first two stanzas of "Opportunity," by the poet Walter Malone:

> They do me wrong who say I come no more
> When once I knock and fail to find you in;
> For every day I stand outside your door
> And bid you wake, and rise to fight and win.
>
> Wail not for precious chances passed away!
> Weep not for golden ages on the wane!
> Each night I burn the records of the day--
> At sunrise every soul is born again!

Malone's message is that each of us gets opportunities every day to be present in our lives, to mine the joy of living. The awakening, I realized when it happened to my dad, was not just for my dad. It was for me, my brother, my sister, my kids, and their kids. And I want to keep giving Dad's gift out. I want to give it to you and your family. And I want to hear about your awakenings, so that we can keep the circle growing.

I hope that this book will lead you to your own awakenings, or to recognize the ones you've already had. And then maybe you'll share it with those in your life. I'm also recording a companion podcast, and I hope you will also find that, so that you can hear the awakenings that others have already shared with me. In some ways, maybe since the pandemic, but maybe even before, many of us have become unmoored from our lives: in them, but not observant of them, and an awakening can *bring you back to your life*.

Your life and your awakenings are miracles, and I hope this book will encourage you to share them with those you love, and maybe even with me, on my podcast. So thank you for finding this book. It means everything to me that I can share my story with you, and I would so love to hear your story too.

Love~

Dan

Chapter 1
Awakening from Dementia

My dad developed dementia in 2005 as a result of a stroke. By the summer of 2015, my dad was in the late stages of dementia and was hospitalized with pneumonia for ten days. It took a lot out of him. He became incontinent and needed to be fed. He would often get agitated and cry like a child in pain (although no one was hurting him) when we shaved him or bathed him. He barely spoke, had no short-term memory, and needed 24-hour care. Prior to this episode, I could take Dad and Mom out to the movies and lunch, but sadly, those special times were no longer possible. And although I still followed my own advice of "acceptance" and "inclusion" (at that point, I still watched TV with my dad, and we would enjoy a meal together at home), I was overwhelmed with sadness.

My father was and *is* my hero. My dad grew up with three older brothers, so he became the protective "older brother" for each of his friends. He was never afraid to take on the local bully. In fact, he was an undefeated boxer in the army, going 26–0.

My father's toughness and drive served him well in life. He turned his street smarts into a successful business and marketing career. He was also a generous man who treated others with respect and kindness. No matter what his lot in life, he showed his appreciation to those kind to him, for example, Dad was always a generous tipper.

My dad was perhaps the most protective of, and most loving toward, his wife and three children. His messages to us growing up—

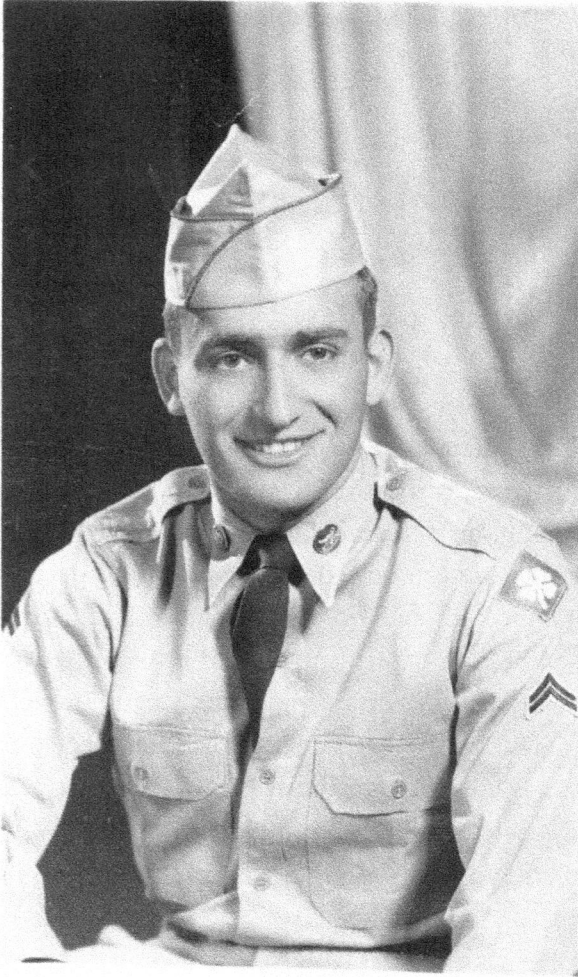

Dad in the Army.

seemingly contradictory but ultimately reasonable—were these: *You can do anything you put your mind to, and as long as you do your best, that's okay.*

My father also had his quirks, which only made him funny and charming, in my view. He never wanted more than "a sliver of cake" and then would eat five slivers. He also had a habit that I think was really old-fashioned, more than anything: he would put a long brown or black sock across his eyes when he took a nap or went to sleep. My father was my best friend, so to see his strong presence deteriorate over time was heartbreaking.

After the pneumonia seemed to steal the last of my father's humanity, he got it again, along with bad hypertension. The hospital had to treat him with a high dose of steroids and antibiotics, because they were afraid the second pneumonia could be the end. During this hospital stay, it seemed as if a switch was flipped, and my dad began to *AWAKE*.

My brother Ken is an internist/cardiologist. One of his partners was Dad's doctor. Ken had admitting privileges at the hospital, so he was present often when Dad was hospitalized. As a result, he spent the most time with Dad.

Besides being my hero, Dad was the single most profound influence in Ken's life as well. Ken describes Dad, before the dementia, as a man who exuded love. He describes the dementia as being insidious at first, before rapidly progressing to a point where Dad hardly recognized us.

Ken witnessed Dad's awakening first. When he looks back on it, it still blows his mind and causes the hair to stand up on the back of his neck. Describing the awakening, Ken said, "He started to become more alert, and then it became like a light switch, 'Hey, I'm back!', and he had full conversations."

When I entered his room, at first I didn't realize what was happening. My dad asked me, "How are you doing?" The importance of what he said didn't dawn on me immediately because my father no longer initiated conversation or spoke in full sentences. He hadn't asked me about my own life or well-being for years. But at first, I didn't realize how huge this was, that he was initiating a normal conversation.

I responded, "I'm okay, Dad."

Then, he said, "You know I love you very much." I suddenly realized my father was much more alert—not quite the man he'd been before his stroke, but he had a strong resemblance to him. I felt my face lift into a wide smile.

My dad smiled back and then asked, "What happened to me?"

I responded, "You have pneumonia. You are being treated and hopefully can go home soon." I realized later that he might have been asking, "Where have I been these past ten years?"

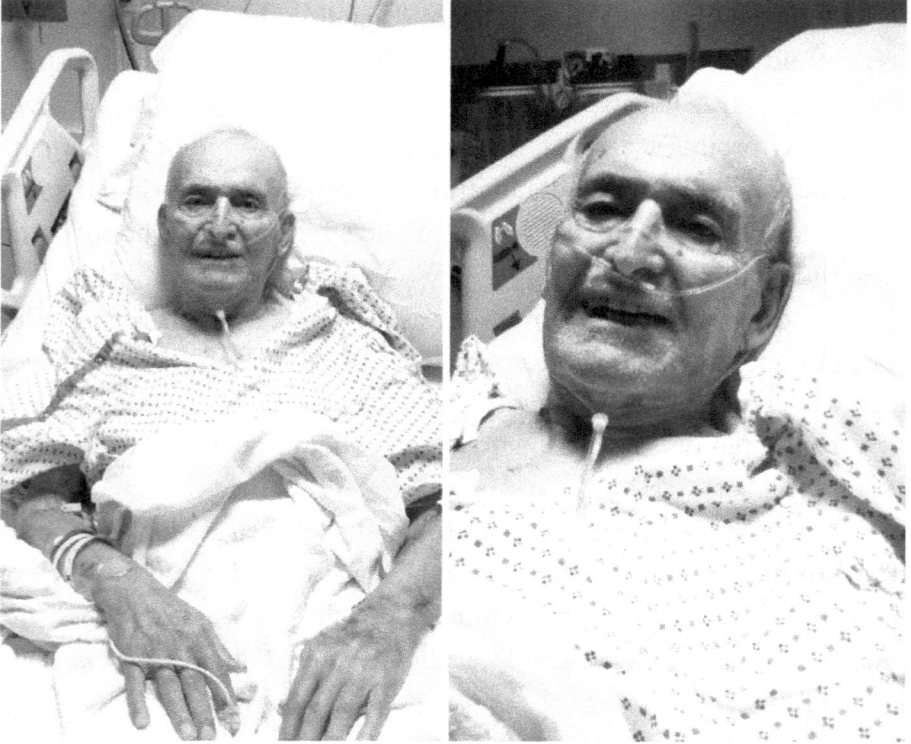

Dad "awake."

My father's awakening continued for two days, and my brother videotaped some of it on the last day. Among the wonderful things we were able to experience:

- My father told my brother it was great to have a son like him and that he was grateful for his children and grand-children. Ken said that to hear that from Dad was unbeliev-able and one of the seminal moments of his life to see his dad come back.

- When we gave him family updates, he'd respond, *"That's interesting,"* or *"That's fabulous."*
- He also asked my sister about her beloved dog, which she had adopted *while* he was in the early stages of dementia. She was moved that he remembered.
- He also joked with us, like when my sister mentioned it was Labor Day, and he quipped, "Yeah, I'm working real hard."
- We also talked with my father about sports, which he loved, and Jewish athletes in particular, which always delighted him because there have been so few famous ones.
- At one point, he told my Mom, "You are the love of my life." After sixty-two years of marriage, I'm sure the words had special meaning for her; in fact, I could see the emotion on her face.
- We also discussed Wayne Chrebet, my father's favorite football player, who overcame unbelievable odds to succeed

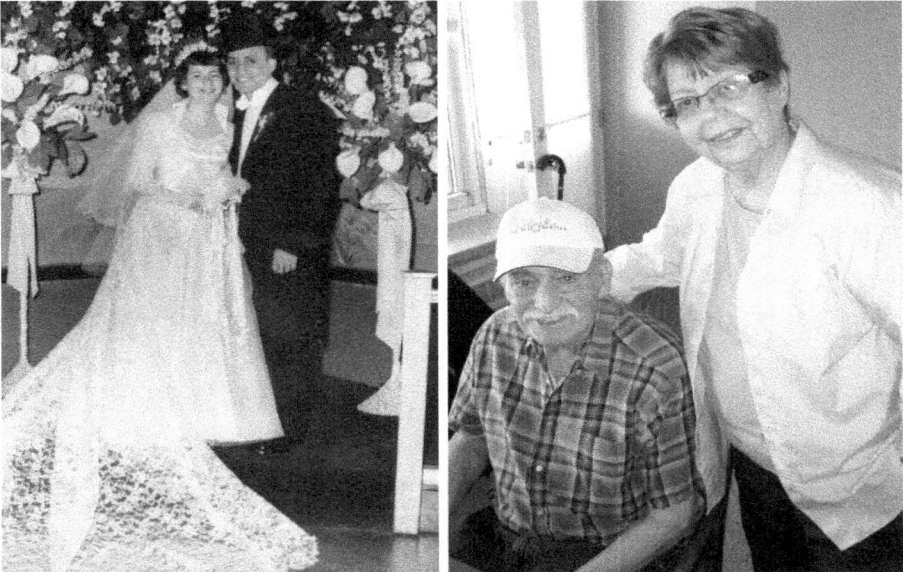

Mom and Dad's wedding photo and (at right) 62 years later.

29

in the NFL. Talking about his own boxing career, my dad said he was underestimated like Chrebet, and so often surprised his opponents. With tears in his eyes, my dad recalled the holiday picture of him and his grandchildren dressed alike in Wayne Chrebet's jersey. He then asked, "What is Chrebet doing now?" I Googled it and told him.

- Perhaps the most remarkable aspect of my dad's awakening was his interaction with my Mom, who lived with him every day and clearly suffered the most from seeing my dad's worsening condition.

- It made us all smile when he wanted to take a nap and asked my mother for the sock for his eyes. I was surprised he remembered he'd used to do that.

- Maybe equally as amazing was when he asked Mom for some money so he could tip the nurses and aides who had been so nice to him. I didn't know how he could possibly have known they had been so nice to him, but my dad wanted to give them a little something to show his appreciation.

If I had to put it in percentages, during the awakening, I would say Dad was 90% of the man I remembered. Ken didn't describe it in percentages but said that the bar was so low and he came back so high. Ken said Dad answered every question correctly.

Sadly, my father's *Awakening* was temporary, and he reverted to his dementia, and it was as bad as ever. Our emotions were mixed— blessed that we had the time with Dad when he was alert, but sad it didn't last. We were filled with questions.

Why did that happen? We hoped there was a medical explanation that could be replicated to bring Dad back. My father's neurologist said he had never seen anything like it in his thirty years of practice. My brother, an internist and cardiologist, theorized at the time that my father had been suffering from *hypoadrenalism*, or a lack of steroids, and when Dad was infused with high doses of steroids, his body and mind temporarily healed, and he became much more alert. More recently, my brother researched the issue again and discovered that steroids can actually have an adverse effect on a dementia patient. If you look today, it seems that in general steroids are not recommended to help with dementia, so maybe the steroids didn't wake Dad up. Ken's most recent explanation is that because Dad's pneumonia got better, there was a change in Dad's neurotransmitters and his dopamine levels. Despite all the theories, Ken said that in all his years of practice, he has never seen anything like Dad's awakening. And when telling the story to his physician colleagues, they confirm having never experienced anything like it in their practices as well.

One thing about having someone in your life experience dementia is that there are so many things about the disease that are just not understood, and cannot be explained well to us, the ones around the person with dementia. I was there, in the room with my dad when he woke up, and I still have trouble understanding how someone suffering with dementia, a *progressive* mental disease with loss of function, can suddenly become more alert.

Maybe it's a miracle? I'm not a religious person and have never given much thought to miracles, but this seems to me to be as logical a conclusion as steroids or dopamine levels reversing an irreversible progressive disease. Miracles don't have to be logical, and a lot about dementia seems illogical, so I'm leaning toward miracle.

Maybe my father was sending his family a message? Besides the expressions of love he was able to give to all of us, maybe there is more meaning to his conversations with us over those days when he had woken up. Dad had been a fighter his whole life, and maybe he wanted to remind us never to underestimate him because he planned to continue to surprise us and fight this disease too, just like the fighter he had been his whole life. That would be easy for me to believe, because my dad always did hang in there and do his best, and I can easily accept that he would fight his way to the surface for one last chance to tell us he loved us.

Could we have recreated what happened to my dad? First, even if there was a medical explanation, treatment would not have been an option because his health was incredibly fragile. Second, if it had been a miracle, and we all prayed for another, miracles don't happen twice. That's what makes them miraculous. Third, we realized that with dementia, it is important to be in the present, the now, as much as possible, so we decided to accept the change in Dad, and cherish it, for as long as it lasted.

My son and daughter were twenty-five and twenty-two when my dad, their grandad, woke up. When they were able to get back and visit my dad, he'd already reverted to his prior mental state. My daughter was overwhelmed with emotion, because she had really been hoping for a chance to be with her grandad as she remembered him, even for a few days. We were able to show my daughter and my son the video my brother had taken, which, honestly, was another blessing. That my brother had thought to record was amazing to me, I'll always be grateful. My daughter got to see her grandfather say, *"I'm very happy just to be here and alive,"* on the video, and it meant so much to her.

I believe Dad was telling us that even in the throes of dementia, *he valued life and wanted to live.* Ken said maybe he was more aware in the dementia than we normally thought. How did he know what hospital he was in when asked, or that one grandchild was in medical school and another in an Ivy League school—events that occurred while he had dementia.

After my dad woke up, and while still in the hospital, he went back to sleep, deep inside himself, and his dementia took control again. When he was well enough to be discharged, he was able to go back home, but he also went home to hospice care.

I asked my brother how he was impacted by Dad's awakening. He said, "As a doctor, it exponentially increases my hope for other patients. Anything is possible. I've seen things that other people would consider miracles. Advances in heart disease, cancer therapies, and more."

I don't think I will ever get over losing my father, or missing him, or feeling robbed, to some extent, by the terrible disease that is dementia. Sometimes dementia feels like the person has died and left their living body behind. I think it makes us realize how much of the person is the mind and spirit, and not the body. But even in my anguish, I found hope. When my father woke up, it showed me he was still in there and wanted to live. It helped all of us reconnect with Dad and connect more deeply with each other, and it changed Dad, even for that brief time, from patient back into *Dad*. It confirmed for me what I had hoped every time I'd had a meal with him, or visited him and my mom, *my dad was in there.*

Note: In the premiere episode of the *Awakenings In Real Life* podcast, my brother Ken and I share this story for anyone who may be interested in putting voices to the narrative.

REFLECT

When I think about what I want for, and from, this book, the first thing I think of is that I want to share it with you. That means I want to give you my story, and, if possible, receive yours. I am adding these thoughts to reflect on so that I think deeply about my story, and maybe you will think about yours, too. And if you feel able, maybe you'll write some thoughts here on the notebook pages throughout, and possibly share them with the people in your life, or send them to me, or both.

When my father woke up from his dementia, I changed. I became a much more reflective person than I was before. I wish I could give you the same experience of having your loved one wake up, but what I can do is to invite you to reflect with me. It's so difficult to take time for yourself during dementia care or caring for anyone with a serious mental or physical illness or disability, but doing so can leave you much more refreshed for your next interaction as caregiver or family member. So I hope you'll take a moment to reflect with me, and I encourage you to write it down, right here, in case you forget later.

When I reflected on those brief days my dad turned back into his old self, I realized that I believe my dad's reversal *was a message, not only for me and our family, but maybe for other family members or caregivers of Alzheimer's/Dementia sufferers; a message of hope that our loved one still appreciated life and wanted to live.*

When you consider your person who is living with dementia or any other mental or physical illness, what signs can you see that they are still enjoying some aspect of being alive? What clues can you spot that the person you love is in there, even if the outside is different? Is there a food they love, a song that perks them up? Take this moment to reflect on your time with your person, and see if you can spot any clues. Let's see if, even with this hard time, we can still find joy, together.

Dan

Add your reflections here.

Chapter 2
I Wish I Could Flip a Switch and Wake Up My Father

To really understand Dad and his dementia journey, it helps to start at the beginning. And while his Awakening was very profound, there were lessons I learned during his journey that I would like to share as well.

In early November 2005, my dad, Herbie, was walking into my brother's medical office when he had a stroke. He was mumbling, and one side of his face was drooping. He couldn't smile. He was bleeding into his brain. Within ten minutes, he was in the ER, and they stopped his bleeding. The quick action saved his life, and he lived another eleven years. Unfortunately, because of the stroke, Dad developed dementia.

Dementia is a general term used to describe a group of cognitive disorders affecting memory, reasoning, thinking, and social skills. It interferes with the daily lives of the individuals who have it. Symptoms include memory loss, confusion, communication issues, not knowing where they are, difficulty completing tasks or problem solving, lack of coordination, anxiety and depression, changes in personality, agitation, and trouble recognizing both loved ones and others.

According to the Mayo Clinic, dementia can be caused by several factors or diseases, including:

1. Alzheimer's disease: The most common cause of dementia, characterized by the buildup of plaques and tangles in the brain.
2. Vascular dementia: Caused by damage to blood vessels in the brain, leading to reduced blood flow and brain cell loss.

3. Neurodegenerative disease: Such as Multiple Sclerosis, Parkinson's disease, and Huntington's disease.
4. Brain trauma: Head injuries like my dad had, or concussions, can damage brain tissue and cause, or increase the risk of, dementia.
5. Other causes, including infections (such as syphilis and HIV), metabolic disorders, and certain vitamin deficiencies.

The Mayo Clinic* also identifies the following as factors that can increase the risk of dementia:

1. Excessive smoking or alcohol use
2. Genetics
3. Lack of physical or mental activity
4. Poor diet
5. Stress
6. Age.

Dementia is typically progressive and gets worse over time. In the beginning, Dad made a great recovery and was able to drive a car again. For the first few years, he had a strong resemblance to himself, even as he slowly deteriorated.

By 2012, Dad was losing his short-term memory. His conversations were shorter, and he was walking with assistance. He needed help getting dressed and washed. My dad could no longer drive.

I am not a doctor who treats Alzheimer's and dementia patients. I am not a professional caregiver. By no means do I profess to be an expert on the subject. In 2012, Mom was Dad's primary caregiver. I was his son who visited often. Is my experience unique? Probably not. Does

*Dementia. (n.d.). Mayo Foundation and for Medical Education and Research. https://www.mayoclinic.org/diseases-conditions/dementia/symptoms-causes/syc-20352013

it differ from other family members of persons with dementia or dementia caused by Alzheimer's disease? Probably not. All I can do is share my experience and hope it resonates with you. It's cathartic for me to write about my experience, and maybe, just maybe, my experience or perspective can help others. But no, I don't have medical advice for you, just, hopefully, comfort in knowing you're not alone on your journey with this disease.

In 2012, I was preoccupied with this thought that kept running through my mind: *I wish I could flip a switch and wake up my father. I know my father is in there.*

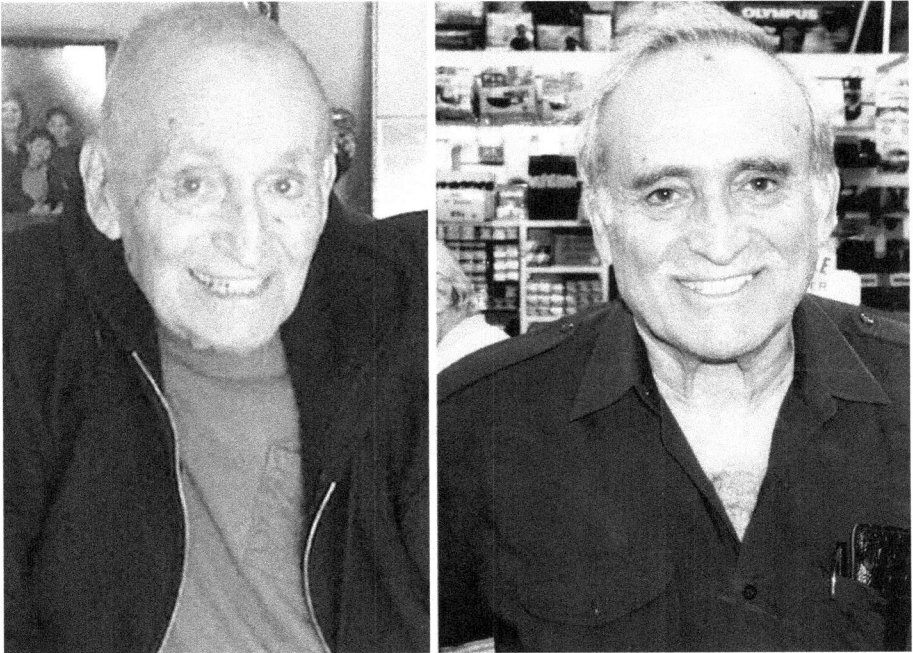

Dad with dementia and (at right) before dementia.

I missed my confidant, my problem solver, my best friend. I missed his big personality, his sense of humor, his guidance, and his enveloping love. We would talk every day, and there was never a conversation we had where he didn't end it with, "I love you to pieces."

As most people know, dementia gets worse over time. It typically runs in "stages." There are seven stages of dementia:

1. No Cognitive Decline – No memory problems; Normal functioning.
2. Very Mild Cognitive Decline – Mild memory loss. No real impact in daily life, but may forget names or places (age-related forgetfulness).
3. Mild Cognitive Decline – but not yet diagnosed as dementia –Difficulty in organizing and planning. Obvious memory issues.
4. Moderate Cognitive Decline – Clear decrease in cognitive function. Confusion about place and time. Problems with simple tasks. Behavioral changes.
5. Moderately Severe Cognitive Decline – Memory loss increases. Help is often needed for daily activities. Person will likely need daily help but can use the restroom and eat on their own.
6. Severe Cognitive Decline – May lose awareness of surroundings. Significant memory loss. Requires assistance with daily activities. May also have major personality, emotional, and behavioral changes.
7. Very Severe Cognitive Decline – Final Stage. Marked by a significant decline in cognitive ability. Will need help with everything, including eating and going to the bathroom. Can't communicate.

In 2012, I was not sure what stage of dementia Dad was in. I was not obsessed with finding out from the doctor either. Honestly, not knowing if it was bad, or very bad, or somewhere in between helped me continue to have hope. We knew Dad was not in good shape; we didn't want to know more than that. I had my interactions with him, and I tried to be "in the moment" with Dad. My suggestion to other

The 7 Stages of Dementia

Stage 1	No cognitive decline
Stage 2	Very mild cognitive decline
Stage 3	Mild cognitive decline
Stage 4	Moderate cognitive decline
Stage 5	Moderately severe cognitive decline
Stage 6	Severe cognitive decline
Stage 7	Very severe cognitive decline

family members or caregivers of sufferers is not to obsess about which stage their loved one is in. It's not going to change things if you know the exact stage and all the possible symptoms that accompany it. It will likely cause you undue hardship and stress. You know what is going on with your loved one, and recognize the deterioration even if it doesn't come with the label. Focus on every day with your person. If dementia has been diagnosed, it is important to be in the moment, to enjoy what you and your person are able to enjoy for as long as your loved one is able to do so. Don't miss out on it by being bogged down in the medical.

At this time, Dad was on a downward trajectory. Luckily for us, he was not depressed or angry, typical symptoms of dementia in later stages, but remained pleasant and calm. At this point, he hardly engaged in conversation, which I think may have been too difficult or taxing for him. Thankfully, he still recognized me, my mother, his kids, grandchildren, and people he knew. I can't tell you how much that meant to all of us. We hoped he would never get to the point where he couldn't remember us.

I often hear people say, when talking about their loved one with Alzheimer's or dementia, how frustrating it is. "My mom repeats things over and over." "My husband forgets what I just told him." It's easy to get short-tempered, "You already told me that," or, "Don't you remember, I just told you that?" Our natural tendency is to challenge someone when they are wrong, or to correct them. I can tell you over and over that your person is not the person you remember when they were perfectly fine, or that it's the fault of the disease, and therefore you should have all the patience possible, but it's still hard when you are in it: when dementia takes over the life of the person you love, it takes over your life, too. When this happens with your loved one over and over, how could you not get upset or exasperated? My advice is not to beat yourself up; you're human. What I suggest is to acknowledge where your loved one is and recognize the behavior as a symptom of the disease without creating confrontation.

Another thing that families do is long for the person's condition six months ago and lament the current condition. "Wasn't he so much better before?" "He remembered more." "She was able to do more." "She needed less help before." But then a friend, whose mother suffered from Alzheimer's and didn't recognize her daughter at the end, gave me great advice boiled down to one word: acceptance. Although it was horrible at the end, my friend would do anything to see her mother in the hospital bed on the morphine drip. Why? *Her mother was still alive.* For me, acceptance meant loving my dad for who he was at each moment in time, and for how much he had meant to me throughout my life, and not only at the end of his. If you're not able to blow off steam with a friend or in some way find your path to acceptance, the frustration you feel will overwhelm the time you have left with your loved one.

In October 2012, my mother traveled to Houston for three days for a party, and my brother, sister, and I took turns staying over and watching my father. Each of us, on consecutive nights, took him to see a movie. The next time we were all together, we spoke about what we had done with Dad. My siblings asked what movie I had taken Dad to see.

"*Argo*" I replied. An audience favorite, *Argo* would go on to win seven Oscars in 2013, including Best Picture.

"I took him to Argo too," my brother said.

My brother and I looked at my sister and, before we could even ask the question, she said, "Yup, *Argo* too."

We burst into laughter at the same time, and I don't think I had laughed that hard in a long time. Dad clearly didn't remember the movie from night to night. On my way home, when I was by myself, I cried like a baby. I vowed to myself that "the Argo experience" for my father would never happen again.

Once, in a dementia support group I belonged to, someone posted something along the lines of the idea that people with dementia leave our world for a world of their own, and to accept that is to let them be, and let them enjoy it.

I understand the sentiment, but I disagree. To me, that is giving up, losing hope, and not accepting your loved one for who they are, but for who they are not. My siblings and I let Dad be in his own world, so it didn't matter if he saw the same movie three days in a row. If we acknowledged and accepted him for where he was in his Dementia battle, we never would have done that and taken him to three *different* movies.

Every other week of 2012, I took Mom and Dad to the movies and lunch. It didn't matter how hard it was to get Dad into and out of the car. It didn't matter that five minutes after the movie, my father didn't remember he'd even gone. It was being with him that counted. And even if he didn't remember on the surface, I always felt like the enjoyable day out lifted him up, emotionally.

I knew that no matter what "stage" my father was in, the essence of who he was remained: a loving man. Although he couldn't express it as he used to, I would see it in his eyes, no matter what.

At the time, I thought about whether I would do anything differently if there came a time when my father couldn't recognize me and the family, and stared at us blankly. That has to be incredibly painful. I hear stories that even when a loved one is in this stage, sometimes there are hints of recognition. And even if that did happen, I knew I would always treat him with love and compassion and as part of this "world." As I see it, to do otherwise would not have been "accepting," so as much as giving up all hope. Everyone knows that, as things stand, dementia is not going to be cured, but the hope should not be for it to be reversed, but for our loved one and ourselves to have the joy of each other as long as we can.

Here are my own definitions of acceptance as a person on a loved one's journey with dementia:

> Acceptance is always being in the moment with your loved one.
> Acceptance is not losing patience with your loved one.
> Acceptance is meeting your loved one where they are at.
> Acceptance is loving yourself no matter your slip-ups or failings.
> Acceptance is having hope even when things seem hopeless.
> Acceptance is loving your loved one unconditionally

I love you to pieces, Dad. When he awakened, Dad showed me that *he was still in there.*

REFLECT

What does it mean to accept? When I talk about acceptance with regards to my dad's dementia, it does not mean giving up when it comes to your loved one suffering from dementia or another debilitating mental or physical illness or disability. I hope we all always strive to do whatever we can to encourage or help our loved one to get better. Sometimes that means taking a moment to rekindle your love for your person. Sometimes, when the disease is very tough, or the person with the illness is agitated or suffering, it's challenging. In my mind, acceptance is loving your person for who they are at the time and loving yourself as well, for trying, for being the best you can be in all the circumstances that affect you in this difficult time.

When you consider your person who is living with dementia or any other mental or physical illness, can you reflect upon those times where you "accepted" the situation and were able to enjoy times with your loved ones instead of getting frustrated or upset, or think of a time where you found some peace while in your tough circumstances? If you think back, you may be able to spot a time, like I have done, where if you could have taken a breath, practiced acceptance, things might have worked better for you and your loved one. It's hard not to judge ourselves, but we all are doing the best we can. Can you note some of your times of acceptance, or some of your times of not being able to accept? Can you imagine for yourself what acceptance would look like, and how it might change your experience and the experience of your loved one?

Let's be in this book together. I accept me, and I accept you. We're hanging in there.

Add your reflections here.

Chapter 3
Freehold Raceway: Love, loss, and Lessons in the most unusual place

I learned that Freehold Raceway permanently closed on Dec. 28, 2024. The news made me sad as this staple of harness racing had been around for over 170 years and was more than just horse racing for me and my family. The news impacted me more than I thought it would, as I had gone there many times over the past thirty-plus years. It wasn't the times we won races, or even the times we lost, that most came to mind, but that the racetrack was a constant in my relationship with my parents, primarily my dad, and later with my kids.

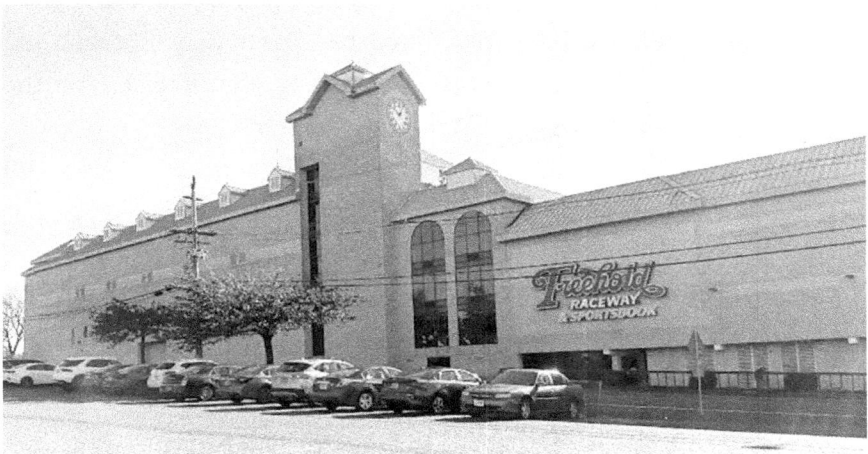

Freehold Raceway, Freehold, NJ.

Dad passed away in 2016, but in May 2005, we gave him a surprise 75th birthday party, attended by his family and close friends. At the party, each family member spoke to Dad about the special bond they had with him. The older grandchildren related stories of playing football, playing catch, and other ways they spent quality time together. For the younger grandkids, they had sleep-overs, went to the arcade, and to Broadway shows with my parents. When it was my then fifteen-year-old son's turn to speak, he said: "While Grandpa takes my cousins to places like the batting cage, that is not what he does with me and my sister. Grandpa takes us to the … racetrack." Those present at the party had a hearty laugh. Little did they know that "The Track," as my Father affectionately called horse racing, played an ongoing role in our interactions with him.

When I was a kid, my dad took me to Roosevelt and Yonkers Raceways during the year and Monticello Raceway in the Catskills during the summer. I was always excited when the race would begin with the booming announcement, "The Marshall Calls the Pacers." Later, when I had kids, we went to Freehold Raceway because it was near my house in New Jersey, the nation's fastest half-mile harness racetrack. While thoroughbred racing features jockeys riding on the backs of horses, in harness racing, horses pull a two-wheeled vehicle (called a sulky) occupied by a driver. Dad liked harness racing because there seemed to be more strategy involved; it was a slower pace than thoroughbreds, and he could handicap the races better.

My son and I started going with Dad to the track around 1995, when my son was five years old. My younger daughter joined us later. My son, Dad, and I went to the track the weekend before my son started first grade. On that day, the moon and stars were aligned as everything went right. Dad was on a huge hot streak. He must have won half the races and won a few hundred dollars or more. We celebrated every victory. Dad told his grandson he could have anything he wanted at the toy store, and my son picked out the biggest LEGO he could find.

On my son's first day of first grade, the teacher asked the students questions to get to know them. She asked them to tell her what they would do if they had $100. My son responded that he would go to Freehold Raceway.

Luckily for my wife and me, we never received that dreaded call from his teacher or the principal. I guessed at the time it was because the local mall was called "The Freehold Raceway Mall." I shared the story with my parents, and we had a good laugh. Early the following week, Dad asked if we could go to the track the upcoming weekend. We never went back-to-back weekends, and I said, "Let's do it another time." He insisted and said it was because he was on a hot streak. So, we went the following Saturday. My son was excited about winning again and getting another huge LEGO. Instead, Dad did not win one race, and we all felt dejected, especially my son, who did not get another toy. I said to Dad that I was sorry we didn't win any races. He winked at me, and I realized that he had lost all the races on purpose.

My dad then turned to my son and said, "Always remember that when you gamble on the horses, you will usually lose money; when you go to the track, *expect* to lose."

Ten years later, as my son finished his speech to Grandpa on his 75th birthday, he added this note: "Grandpa, I know you now like to go to the casino, play blackjack and poker, and all that fun stuff. You're allowed to go, don't get me wrong, but I have to tell you something . . . *expect* to lose." Again, the crowd laughed. It suddenly dawned on me at that moment that my son, who was used to getting a participation trophy even if his team lost, had learned from my dad that life is not always a bed of roses.

From 1996 to 2005, we went to the track with my dad two or three times a year. It was always a fun time. Mom would sit reading a book. We had fast food and ice cream. We bonded as a family. I think it was also the place my daughter learned to root for a team, watching grown men shout for their horse to win. It was so cute hearing her shout her horse's number or name out as loud as she could among a chorus of grown men.

Each time we went, Dad felt particularly strong about one horse in one race. He had become a good handicapper over the years. As he studied the racing form, he would circle certain information he read there, like:

- The horse's odds of winning
- Where the horse finished in its last five races
- How fast it ran
- Track conditions
- Its competition, among other things.

In the race, the horse he selected was typically, but not always, the favorite, meaning it had the best odds of winning, but it also meant it would pay the least. On these races, he usually won six out of ten times.

And then, in November 2005, Dad had a stroke. He bled into his brain. Within ten minutes, he was in the ER, and they stopped the bleeding. The quick action saved his life, and he lived another 11 years. Unfortunately, because of the stroke, Dad developed dementia. Dementia progressively worsens over time. In the beginning, Dad made a great recovery, and still loved to go to the track, and we still went as a family.

Dementia has seven stages of cognitive decline. By 2012, Dad was losing his short-term memory. Even as I could see it progressing, I didn't judge the evolution of his dementia the way his doctors did. I know this may sound odd, but I had a very tangible way of determining Dad's dementia. Each year, I observed his ability to read the horse racing form. As each year went by, he circled fewer and fewer items on the race form. That's how I knew the disease was changing my dad: he was losing his ability to work the racing form.

By 2013, my father's dementia had progressed to the point where he had little short-term memory and needed help taking care of himself. He was still amiable, and not angry or depressed, though those are typical symptoms of dementia. At that point, he hardly started a conversation, and when he was engaged, he usually responded with few words. Fortunately, he still recognized his immediate family, which meant the world to all of us. Despite his illness, Dad still asked to go to the track. Maybe it was embedded deep in his memory, but he knew it was something that he liked. I knew that soon after we left the track, Dad would forget that we had even gone. That didn't matter to me, because at that moment, while the horses were running, he was present and knew what was going on. He could still celebrate our wins. By that time, the only thing Dad circled on the racing form was the odds of each horse winning.

Over the next two years, Dad's dementia continued to worsen. It was much harder to take him out of the house. In 2015, out of nowhere, he asked to go to the track. I knew that three minutes after he asked me to go, he would forget what he had asked. I wasn't sure if he could even enjoy the experience when he was there. It was hard to tell what he could and could not process. It wouldn't be easy to get him there either. My parents lived two hours away in New York. I would have had to do a lot of driving in one day. But, the track was something Dad loved, so I decided to make it happen and include him.

Dad passed away in 2016. At his funeral, my son spoke and relayed the story of the last time we went to Freehold Raceway as a family. He said, "Grandpa could no longer read the racing program or contemplate the odds for each horse. I think he was just picking numbers. On the first race, he picked horse number seven to win. Grandma looked up from her book and said, 'He doesn't know what he is doing; that horse is the biggest long shot in the race.' I jumped right in and said, 'Grandma, never question Grandpa when he feels strongly about a horse in a particular race.' My dad doubled down and said, 'When Dad says a horse is going to win, it usually does.'

"Although our defense of Grandpa was plainly tongue in cheek, we were going to make a bigger bet than usual. Our horse was losing most of the race as predicted, but then out of nowhere, he started to make his move, passing horses down the stretch and pulling out a win by a nose. Grandpa exhibited no emotion during the race or when our horse crossed the finish line first, but a huge smile appeared when we told him his horse had won. I'm so happy we went to the track that day. It's a memory I'll always treasure."

This horse made a great comeback, just like Dad did many times over the years he had dementia. There were several occasions when he was in the hospital, and we were told he wasn't going to make it through the night, but by morning, he'd miraculously recovered. Dad was a fighter his whole life, a great boxer in the service, and he became a successful businessman without a college education.

We learned never to count Dad out, because he had an incredible will to live. My kids also learned about resiliency and how precious life and certain moments can be. Most important to me, that despite Dad's circumstances, we *included* him in this outing and have a lasting memory.

REFLECT

Can you reflect with me on your loved one and your journey with them? If so, please feel free to write this book with me, and include your thoughts below.

Our final trip to the racetrack wasn't enjoyed by my dad like the other trips had been, but it is a lasting memory for my family and me. Dementia or any other serious mental or physical illness is painful for the whole family, and after your loved one has moved on from this life, you may feel that you missed out on opportunities to spend time with them.

Can you think of something you've done with your person since he or she developed their sickness or disability that you're glad you included him/her in? Take a moment to reflect on and remember how it affected your loved one, you, and any other people you included. Thanks for taking the trip to the track with me.

Add your reflections here.

PART 2

Dad's Journey With Mental Illness and Therapy

Author's Note

My dad's dementia was a long journey. He had it for over ten years. In the early days, my dad was closer to his normal self, and as the disease progressed, he would often become buried under the illness. Sometimes he was hale and hearty, and sometimes he was incredibly frail. It was a disorienting experience for my dad, but for all of us who loved him too.

I often felt I had no time, between my dad's health, working a job, and being a father, to think and wrap my mind around what we were in the middle of. Because my dad lived so much in the present then, I tried to do so too. One day, in the midst of this period, I wrote a post on the website Medium about my dad. With no real effort to promote it, it found a lot of readers. A lot of people were also going through the same thing, or had been through it. I was enormously grateful for the connections, because I needed to know we weren't alone, but I didn't really have the time or energy to seek connection. After I lost Dad, I kept going back to those responses, to feeling so grateful for the connection, and decided that I wanted to turn the experience into a full book, but I didn't want the book to be just a sad story about dementia.

My dad, Herbie, was an interesting, complex, and unique person before dementia hid his light away. The more I reflected on the stories others had sent to me, and on my time with my dad in happier days, primarily before the dementia, I realized that to get a full picture of Dad, and a full picture of the toll of dementia, I wanted to reflect on what I knew of him, and what my dad's life had been like before I came along, and after I came along. This path also opened up new ways to reflect on the dementia journey. I hope the stories of the broader life of my dad, Herbie, and me, his son Dan, will continue to open up reflections for you too.

Chapter 4
Growing Up

In order to have a more complete picture of my dad and the man he became, it's important to know a little of his background. My father, Herbie, was born on May 5, 1930, soon after the Great Depression began. He was the youngest of four brothers, Sammy, Benny, Stanley, and Herbie. Sammy was twelve years older than my dad, Benny ten years older, and Stanley, four years older. They were born to immigrant parents, my Grandpa Joe, and Grandma Sadie. Grandpa Joe immigrated from Lithuania, and Grandma Sadie from Russia.

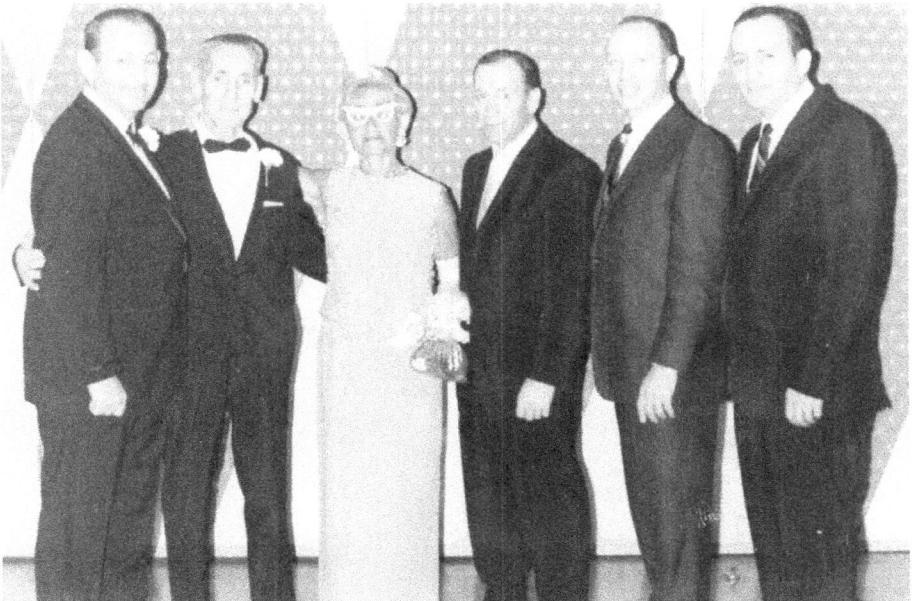

Dad's family.

Grandpa Joe was a very handsome man and spoke seven languages: English, Russian, Polish, German, Lithuanian, Yiddish, and Hebrew. Grandma Sadie was quite the character. She was catered to by her sons, especially my Uncle Benny. Uncle Benny never married and lived with and took care of Grandma his whole life, until she passed. She wore a blonde wig until the day she died in 1981. If you asked her, she considered herself to be a real beauty.

My brother likes to tell the story of how he went to pick Grandma up one time at her apartment building in Woodhaven, Queens. He parked his car, passed some people outside her building, and went to get Grandma, but when he got to her apartment, she wasn't there. When he came back downstairs, he saw Grandma fully dressed, in all her glory. He told Grandma: "I went to the apartment, and you weren't there."

She responded in her Polish accent, "I've been standing outside the whole time."

My brother said, "Well, I must've missed you because you look like a teenager." My Grandma laughed and would tell that story over and over. In her mind, he wasn't kidding.

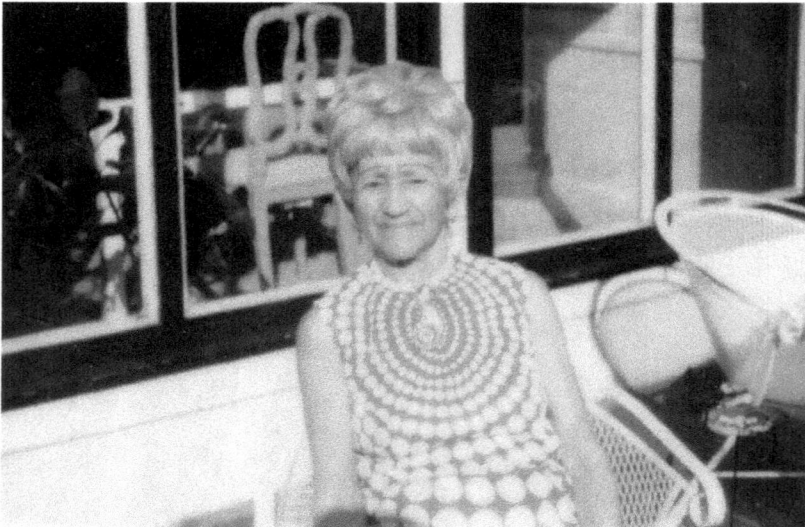

Grandma Sadie.

I remember one time visiting my Grandmother in her apartment in Florida in the 1970s, or as she said it, My-am-eee-Beech!" She was watching soap operas, or what she called her "stories," on a small black-and-white television. I felt so bad that I called up my dad and said, "You have to get Grandma a color TV." My dad agreed, and sent her one from Sears the next week. Grandma got so invested in her "stories" that when she got worried about a character, she would have Uncle Benny call the TV station to make sure everything was going to be okay.

I remember going to a movie with my parents, brother and sister, and my grandparents. We went to see an old movie starring Moishe Oysher, who was an American cantor, recording artist, and a theater, film, and Yiddish actor. It was an old Yiddish film. I also remember Grandpa playing us the song, "My Yiddishe Momme." It's something that sticks with me to this day.

Although I've heard many stories of my dad growing up, a lot of it had to do with him and his brothers fighting with others. They grew up in Williamsburg, Brooklyn, and were tough "Jews." They stood up for themselves and didn't take any crap. I didn't hear a lot of other stories of what it was like for them growing up at home. I always knew my dad was a fast eater. That's because growing up with three older brothers, if he didn't reach for the food quickly, there would be no food left. I also learned that the best part of the steak was the meat on the bone. So, I always wondered why, when my Mother served us steak, my dad and older brother always reached for the meat still on the bone, and I got the heart of the steak.

I always joked that everything "different" or "off" that happened to me occurred because I was the "deprived middle child." For example, why do my siblings eat a variety of foods, and I'm a picky eater? My brother was the firstborn and got all the glory and love associated with his position in the birth order of the family. I came next, three years later, another son. My sister arrived next, six years after me. In a family that was predominately male, this was a joyous event, and she became the princess of the family. When I look back at certain family portraits, you will see my dad, my mom, my brother, my sister, and my right ear lobe.

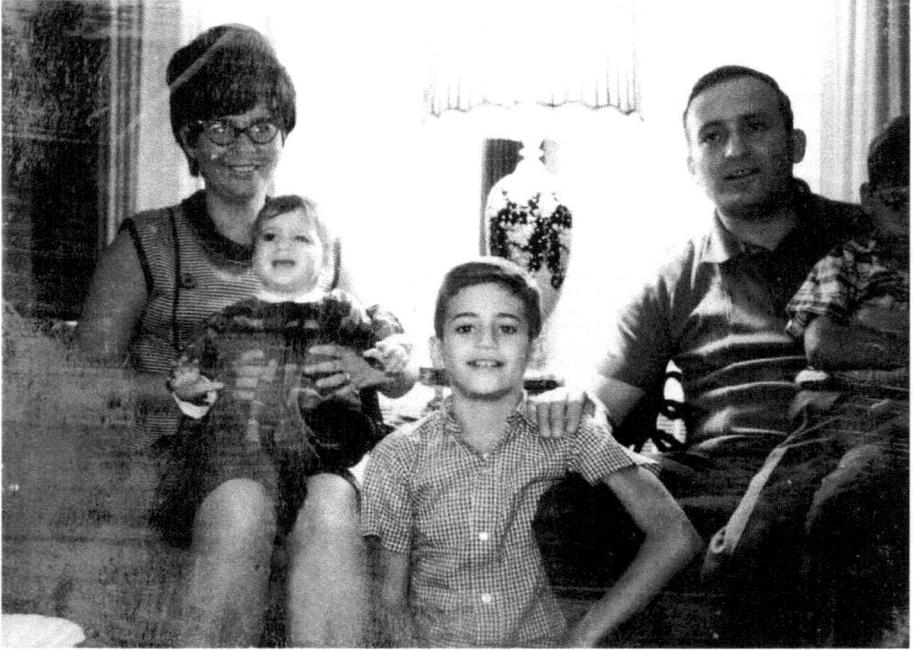

Dan, the middle child.

While I say this tongue-in-cheek, maybe there is something to "Middle Child Syndrome." But my dad would remind me that he was the youngest of four boys, so not to complain too much.

One of the things I learned from my dad about growing up in his home is that his parents weren't the warmest and most loving people. They rarely showed love in a demonstrative way. I also learned that Grandma Sadie was sometimes mean to Grandpa Joe. As I said, my grandpa was a handsome man who spoke multiple languages. I think she might have been jealous of him. She could also be mean to Uncle Benny. She would tell him, "You are worthless like your father." I'm sure this contributed to Benny never getting married, and was maybe why Benny never left home. Dad and Benny were incredibly close their entire lives. When they were younger, they slept in the same bed. I'm sure Grandma's poor treatment of Benny deeply affected my dad as well, because of his love for his brother.

I know my dad loved Grandma Sadie because he also catered to her his whole life. In fact, my Mom knew that she could not challenge Grandma Sadie no matter what she did, and that she had to know their place. My mom would tell me that she let a lot of things go when it came to Grandma Sadie. If they challenged Grandma, it wouldn't have gone over well with her sons.

My dad had a complicated relationship with his mother. He called her every day, and I heard him many times on the phone with his mother saying, "Ma, Ma, give me a break," and things similar to that.

I'm sure Dad's home life caused him a lot of angst as a young man. However, Dad did something at the age of twenty, in 1950, that was not typically done by the youth of his generation. He went to a therapist to get help, and this man helped him immensely. Dad saw this therapist throughout his life. In fact, to honor the therapist, my father made up a plaque of all his therapist's sayings or advice and hung it on the wall in our apartment.

With the help of therapy, Dad was able to overcome many of his childhood demons and become a loving parent to his own wife and children. Of course, he wasn't perfect, but he hugged and kissed us often, and told us we could accomplish anything we wanted in our lives. He was very present in our lives. He also helped my mom tremendously. She grew up in a home with parents who loved her, but they were not demonstratively loving toward her. So, as a result of my dad's influence, my mom showed us, her children, lots of love. My mom also rubbed off on my dad in many ways as well. She was college-educated, while my dad was not, and we grew up knowing that an education was very important.

My father's advocacy for therapy was passed down, as I have had individual therapy, and there were times when we had family therapy as well. While there are different schools of therapy, a good therapist can be very effective. I have been in therapy for over twenty years, and I find it to be extremely helpful. Sometimes having an independent, objective third-party listen and hear you can help you navigate life's obstacles. It can be tremendously useful to one's mental health. I am a big advocate for therapy.

To me, it's a shame that going to a psychologist, social worker, or psychiatrist still has a stigma for a portion of our society. Why is it fine to go to an orthopedist when we break a leg or an internist when we have the flu, but seeing a counselor for mental issues is sometimes frowned upon? My father, to his credit, was ahead of his time by recognizing that he needed help at an early age, and that advocacy has been passed down to me.

REFLECT

Were you surprised to read that my grandmother sometimes wasn't the nicest person? That my dad went to therapy, and so do I? One of the things my dad's dementia made me come to terms with is that not all the people in our lives are kind or treat us as we would like them to. I also learned from my dad that a person is a body, mind, and spirit, and that any one of those parts of you can sometimes need or benefit from assistance. No one should face stigma for which of those three parts they need help with.

There are, then, a few choices for reflection here:

If a person in your life is living with dementia or another mental illness, what is their impact on your life? Is it positive, negative, or somewhere in between?

When you consider getting help in life, is that something you do easily, or is it difficult to ask?

Do you see a person as a body, mind, and spirit? With yourself, how do you honor each of your three parts?

Take this moment to reflect on one of those thoughts and tell me what you learned. Caring for someone with dementia or any mental illness can be very lonely. By doing these reflections, we can connect.

Add your reflections here.

Chapter 5
Dementia Cured My Dad's OCD

Despite Dad's willingness to participate in therapy to improve himself, he suffered from obsessive compulsive disorder (OCD) his whole life. I don't think he was treated for OCD by his therapist, as this was never something he ever mentioned to the family growing up, nor do I know how advanced the diagnosis and treatments were for OCD when he was younger. We all knew he had some "quirks," even though he did a good job hiding them from his children. Dad was not officially diagnosed with OCD until his late sixties, and didn't get specific treatment until that time. This was a man who had a very outgoing personality, and who was demonstrably loving to his family and close friends. He was also street smart and a very successful businessman.

Yet, he struggled with OCD his entire life, and this affected the people around him, primarily my mom.

OCD is characterized by intrusive thoughts and compulsive behaviors. These invasive thoughts and fears lead to repetitive behaviors and rituals to try and ease the obsessions. Most people are probably familiar with the compulsive hand washer, for example. The rituals can manifest themselves in many different ways. Many people may have obsessive qualities, like being a compulsive cleaner, but that doesn't mean they suffer from OCD.

When I was a kid, and then a teen, I knew that Dad had his idiosyncrasies, but I didn't know it as OCD. My father used to ask me all the time, "What did my friend Jay use to throw a ball?"

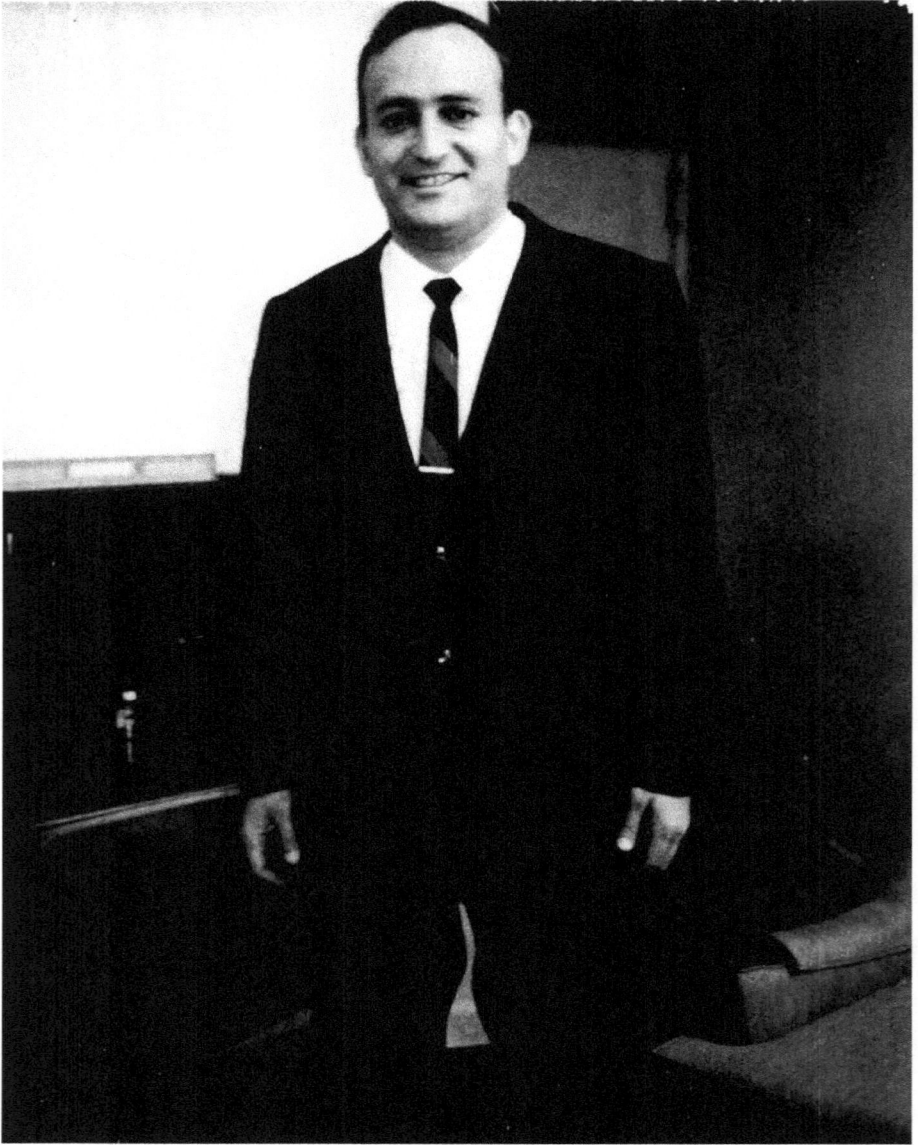

Dad, businessman.

I would respond and say, "He's a lefty."

Not satisfied, Dad would point to his hands and say, "Which one?"

I would then respond, "He uses his left hand." One of my dad's compulsions was to hear the word *hand*. If you could say hand, he wanted you to say it. He also didn't like to see numbers, and he always had the numbers covered in the car or on the clock radio in his bedroom. Dad's OCD also meant he would not go in or near a hospital. He would purposely change directions or go on a detour just to avoid passing by a hospital.

The person who was most affected by my dad's OCD was my mom. Outwardly, my father seemed like the most social guy. When he was with other people, he commanded the room with his sense of humor and personality. However, later in life, my mom would tell me that a lot of times, as a result of his OCD, Dad didn't want to socialize, so they wouldn't go out often. This truly affected my mom as she liked to go out with friends. My mom also said that, typically, my dad's friends were on the quiet side, and very rarely did he have friends that had big personalities like himself. She said this was also part of his OCD. He also did not like to travel much, and although my parents did go on some trips together, eventually my mother took to traveling with friends or my sister.

Despite his OCD, Dad never gave in to the fear when taking care of his family. We grew up in the Warbasse Apartments, which was a middle-income development in Brooklyn, New York, consisting of five buildings with three sections of twenty-three floors each. We were right across the street from Trump Village, owned by Fred C. Trump. Trump Village was also middle-income, but I always viewed it as slightly more luxurious than Warbasse. Trump Village also had seven buildings. There was also Luna Park, a lower-middle-income development con-sisting of five buildings. Growing up in that neighborhood, there were many friends to play with.

I grew up at a time when there was practically no protection for children playing. Most playgrounds were made of concrete and did not have rubber mats or cut-up tires to protect us if we fell. We had monkey bars, and if you fell off, you sometimes broke your leg or arm. We played all kinds of sports growing up, and I had no concern for my body. If we were playing slap ball, a kind of baseball with a rubber ball, and I had to dive to make the catch, I would do so without any concern for how I landed. Most of the time, I landed on concrete and had bruises and scrapes to show for it. I also loved ice cream, and I remember this one time when I tripped while having a chocolate ice cream cone, and although my elbows and knees were scraped and bloody, the ice cream cone remained intact. I had my priorities straight.

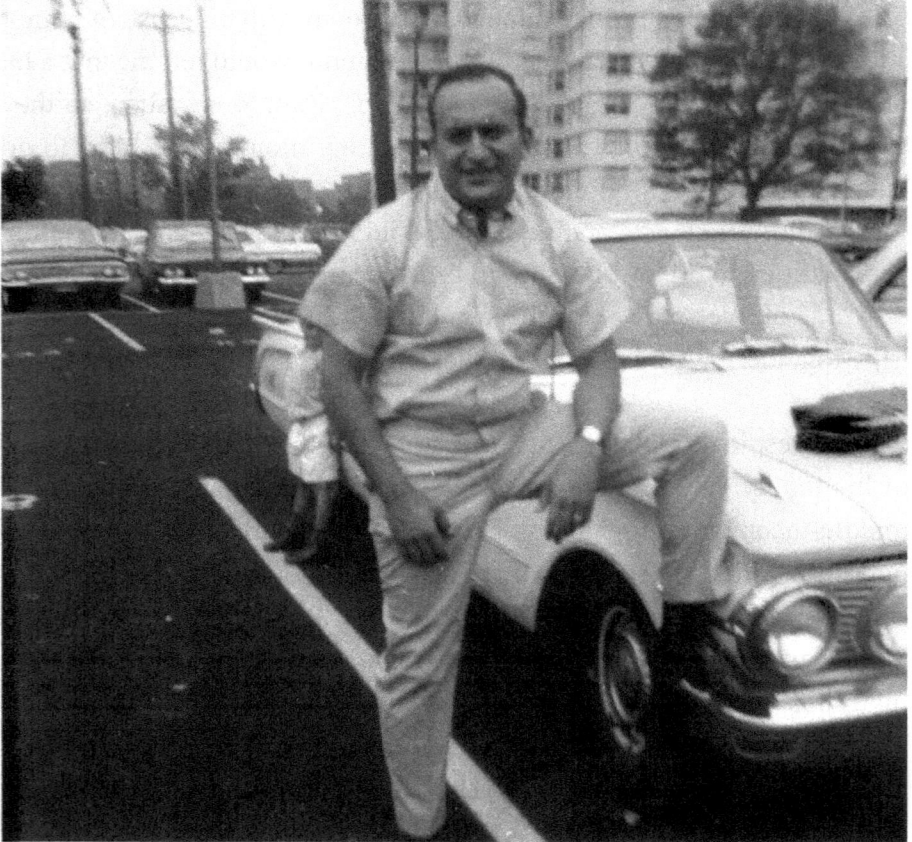

Dad at Warbasse Housing, Brooklyn, NY.

I was very accident-prone when I was young and had more stitches than I can count. We lived on the fourteenth floor in a three-bedroom apartment with one and a half baths, a living room, and a foyer. We never went into the living room or sat on the couch covered in plastic. We all gathered in the smallest room in the house, the foyer, while we watched TV. One night, my parents were sitting in the foyer. They could hear a low wail coming from the hallway. As the scream started to get louder and louder, they realized that it was coming from someone coming up in the elevator. When the scream was very loud, and they could hear crying as well, my mom turned to my dad and said, "Herbie, get your coat on, you have to take Danny to the hospital." And despite his OCD, we made many visits to the emergency room, followed by a stop for a toy or an ice cream on the way home.

When I was eleven years old, I got hit by a car crossing the street on the way back to school after lunch. I was sent to Coney Island Hospital in Brooklyn, and although I didn't break any bones, I chipped some teeth, and my face and body were bruised and battered. My face was so bloody that when the blood dried, it was a frightful sight to see. When it was time for me to go home, and I looked at myself in the mirror, I fainted.

Despite my dad's aversion to hospitals, when I was there overnight, there was nothing that was going to stop him from visiting me. I remember him walking into the room, looking at me and saying, "At least you didn't hurt your nose." I let out a big laugh when he said it, and that made me feel better. You see, in my family, my dad and my brother had the more pronounced nose, and I had my mom's smaller and therefore, my parents thought, nicer nose.

After my dad's stroke and the resulting dementia, *his OCD disappeared*. Was this some medical breakthrough that should be reported to the American Medical Association? Probably not. In this case, we were trading a mental illness that affected my dad's life, but something he could live with, for an illness that would eventually lead to his demise. I guess if it were the other way around, it would really be significant. I know it's a stretch to use the word "cured," but my dad's OCD did stop after his stroke.

As mentioned, Dad's OCD was not classified until he was in his sixties. At the time, one of the ways OCD was managed was to give it a name. It allowed the patient to find a distinct way to separate himself from the condition, allowing the patient to see intrusive thoughts and compulsions as a part of their brain that is not working properly. This is different from that part of their brain that is functioning normally. The lesson the therapist hoped to share with the patient was that OCD behaviors were not the real patient, but a part of the brain that was not working as it was supposed to.

If Dad's therapist did this exercise with him, I can only surmise that Dad would name the OCD something along the line of "annoying" or "controlling," because that part of his brain drove him to do things Dad didn't want to do. Knowing Dad's sense of humor, he might also have named the OCD "J-E-T-S, *Jets, Jets, Jets*," because Dad was a long-suffering New York Jets football fan, and that part of his brain also caused him to suffer. The OCD sufferer knew that there was something wrong in the brain, *without the stigma of feeling that there's something wrong with the patient.* It was "annoying" or "controlling," and that was the real problem, not my dad.

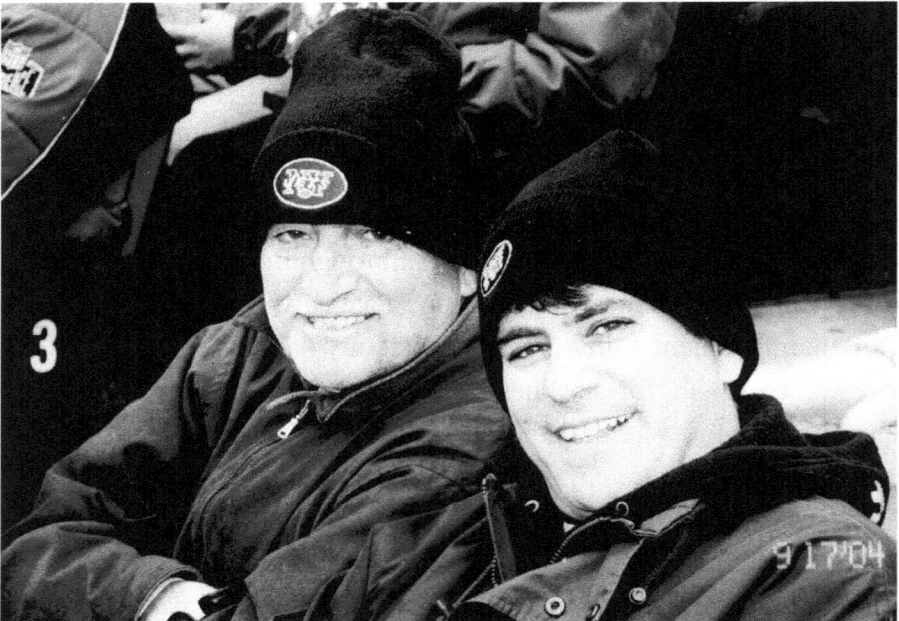

Dan and Dad at a Jets game, one year prior to his stroke.

Wouldn't it be great if all mental illness could be thought of as something wrong with the brain and not the person? OCD is caused when there is a misfiring of the circuits in the brain. It actually has to do with the serotonin levels in the brain being off. Depression is also caused when the serotonin levels in the brain misfire. That's why the same type of drugs, called SSRIs (Selective Serotonin Reuptake Inhibitors) treat both OCD and depression by regulating serotonin levels. The best type of treatment for OCD is a combination of the right medication and behavioral therapy.

The thing about OCD is it's a lifetime affliction, and the person who has it can best cope with it by learning to manage it. For my dad, when he started exhibiting dementia, his OCD symptoms practically stopped. It was as though, among the many things that Dad was forgetting, he was also forgetting his compulsion to hear the word hand, or his need to avoid being anywhere near a hospital. In many ways, as his dementia continued and worsened, Dad's life became less complex, even as his family's life became more complex due to Dad's new needs. For me, OCD wasn't weird; it was just part of my dad's brain that was off. A great guy, and a vulnerable human.

REFLECT

My dad's OCD was really just a part of my dad's brain that was not working properly, not the man himself. It hardly ever interfered with him being my dad, and it never took over from everything else he was. When people get dementia or other mental illness, they can become so different from who they were that it is hard to think of them as who they are, a person with a problem, and easier to think of them simply as the problem itself. Another way to put it is, do we say a person is disabled, or that they're someone who has a disability? The second way takes a little longer to get out of our mouths, and we have to think about what we say before we say it, but that small effort changes a person from a walking disease to a regular person who also has a challenge. Wouldn't it be great if every person's mental illness could be named, so there would never be the stigma associated with the mental illness and a person could get the best treatment possible.

When you consider your person who is living with dementia or another mental illness, has it been easy or difficult to separate the person from the illness? Have you ever gotten a diagnosis for yourself and felt more like a disease and less like a person? Do you have any ideas on how we can help people who have chronic conditions be treated as people first, and conditions second?

I would love to hear your ideas. Take this moment for yourself to reflect on one of those thoughts and share your ideas. Your ideas will be different from anyone else's because of your experiences, and they're incredibly valuable.

Add your reflections here.

_____

_____

_____

_____

_____

_____

_____

_____

_____

_____

_____

_____

_____

_____

_____

_____

_____

_____

_____

_____

_____

_____

_____

_____

_____

_____

_____

_____

_____

_____

PART 3
Family Stories

Author's Note

Some of the stories that follow are based on firsthand knowledge. Others were told to me by sources... mostly reliable: my father and family. Before my dad was my dad, he was Herbie, the youngest of a family of four boys. He grew up in Brooklyn, New York, and he had three tough older brothers and a very tough mother who was both self-important and sometimes cold and demanding toward her family.

The effects of our family reverberate down through the generations. But even as my dad lived with his childhood family and their influences on his life, he also reflected on that, and made conscious changes in his own adult life to turn away from some of those influences. I don't think he ever had a grudge against his upbringing. He cherished it, but he was also the extraordinary person who could see the need to make changes, even as he cherished what had been. In his life, he was demonstrably loving and protective of his family. I think that I am a very reflective person, and I think I got that as one of many gifts from my father.

Chapter 6
How to Handle a Bully

I'm not exactly sure why, but there was a lot of "fighting" in my dad's family. He and his three older brothers grew up in Williamsburg, Brooklyn, way before Williamsburg became hip and cool as it is thought of today. They were a different generation. Maybe it's because they all served in the military, but the fighting started earlier in their lives. What I think all these fights had in common was that, usually, in the stories we were told, the brothers were fighting because they were standing up to a bully. The brothers, in the stories that were told to me, were the good guys. I still think of them that way today, with pride.

I heard a story that my Uncle Sam, twelve years older than my dad, had an "incident" when he was in the military. As the story goes, another soldier was "riding" my uncle pretty hard, repeatedly calling him a "Kike." Kike is a derogatory slur used for Jewish people. It is highly offensive and meant to denigrate and insult Jewish people. After continued harassment, my uncle eventually decked this soldier. My uncle faced no consequences from this fight and was clearly standing up to this bully.

If you're not Jewish, you may not have an understanding that Jewish people have often faced things like Uncle Sam faced, simply for being Jewish. Sam was simply trying to serve our country honorably, but some of his fellow soldiers thought he was somehow less because of his heritage. Jewish people don't all look alike, but if you have certain characteristics, people will make assumptions, and people have long made assumptions about Jewish people. We are not the only ones. Many people from Europe have faced discrimination for being Irish, Italian, Polish, Romanian, to name a few, and people with ancestry from other parts of the world, especially when it makes them look noticeably different, such as those from Asian, Pacific, or African nations, have also had to deal with negative stereotypes being made about them. Being told about my Uncle Sam's experience from the time I was a boy has always helped me try to look for similarities, connections between myself and those different from me. Hating those differences is damaging and upsetting to the hater and the one hated. We could all lose our loved ones to old age, disease, dementia, accidents, and my personal reflection on that is that we really do not have time to spare for worrying about differences, being afraid of them, or actively hating them.

Growing up with tough older brothers, Dad followed in their footsteps and became the protective "older brother" for his friends. One of the most legendary stories, according to my father, that my dad shared with us happened when he was seventeen. Dad and a group of friends had just finished shooting pool and were heading down the narrow staircase to the street below. Heading up to the billiard hall was the toughest seventeen-year-old kid in the neighborhood and his friends. (I'll call him Jimmy here. Jimmy was rumored to be the son of a prominent "wise guy.") Jimmy would not give way to anyone, and, going up the stairs, he aggressively knocked into my dad's best friend, Jerry. When my father asked Jimmy why he had to do that, Jimmy promptly took off his belt, swung it as hard as he could so that the belt buckle smashed onto the top of my father's head. My dad told me he saw stars and said he never felt such pain in his life. He did not run. Instead, he shook it off, squared his shoulders, and proceeded to kick the living crap out of Jimmy. Jimmy needed medical attention afterwards... Weeks later, my dad and Jimmy crossed paths in the street. Preparing for a fight, my father said he gritted his teeth and clenched his fists. Instead of getting into a fight, Jimmy just walked past, nodding at my father as he went by. It was almost as if Jimmy was showing my father some respect for standing up to him. Many years later, my father was reading a book about the top hitmen in America. On the list was Jimmy. And while Jimmy may have had his share of victims in his life, my father and his friends were not one of them.

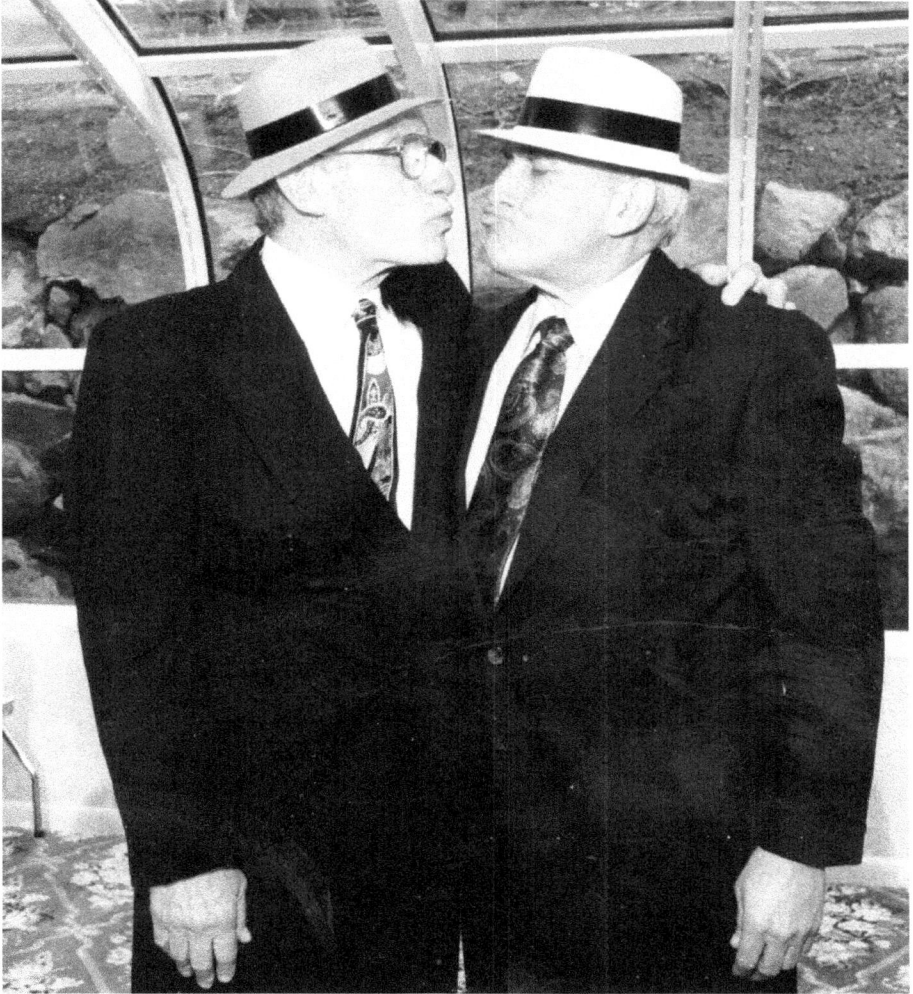

Dad and Jerry later in life.

Dad was never afraid to take on a bully. When he was a little older, he was an undefeated boxer in the US Army. He was smaller, so he fought as a welterweight, but even among the other welterweight boxers, he was underestimated by his opponents, and he took advantage of that by defeating them all, because my dad was tough and a fighter.

My dad was very protective of his children. One time when my brother was in religious school, a bunch of the kids decided to throw prayer books out the window for fun. The Rabbi falsely accused my brother Ken of being a ring leader of the incident, and grabbed him and shook him to try to scare him physically into telling "the truth." As you might expect, my father went up to the religious school to "talk" to the Rabbi. My dad solved problems ninety-nine percent of the time with just his words, but in this negotiation, he threatened to use the same skills he had used on Jimmy as a boy. My dad told the Rabbi that if he ever touched his son again, he would end up out the window himself. Suffice it to say, the Rabbi never touched my brother again. Many kids in a situation like that, where a rabbi, or maybe a nun, or a teacher, accused them of something they hadn't done, back in the days of my childhood, would have gone home to a punishment from their dads. Not in my family. Dad always listened to us, and always believed we were the ones telling the truth, unless the accuser could provide evidence he was wrong. It made my home a very nurturing place to grow up in.

My siblings and I grew up in a different generation from my parents. We were taught to try to solve our problems with our words and not our fists. In fact, we grew up with the greatest problem solver, Dad, who seemingly could accomplish anything with anyone by talking things out.

At my dad's 75th birthday party, my brother's speech consisted primarily of three stories involving my dad. I'll tell one here. When my brother was sixteen, he was coming home from his first date outside of the neighborhood. The date had gone well, and he was happy as he walked home. Suddenly, he was attacked by two neighborhood kids. We never knew exactly why they picked on him, but can only surmise that he was different to them, one of the *smart kids,* and, as such, he appeared a weak, easy target that night. One of the kids put a knife to my brother's throat. My brother was very fast, escaped from the bullies, and ran to our fourteenth-floor apartment, screaming in fear.

When he entered the apartment, he told Dad the story. My dad stopped my brother at the door. "Son, you never run, ever. You go back down there right now and kick their butts." My father's immediate reaction was that my brother had to stand up for himself and fight. And it couldn't wait. It had to be that night. He didn't want my brother to get into fights, but he also didn't want him to live his life afraid of bullies. Bullies, my father knew, are inevitable, but being afraid of them wasn't.

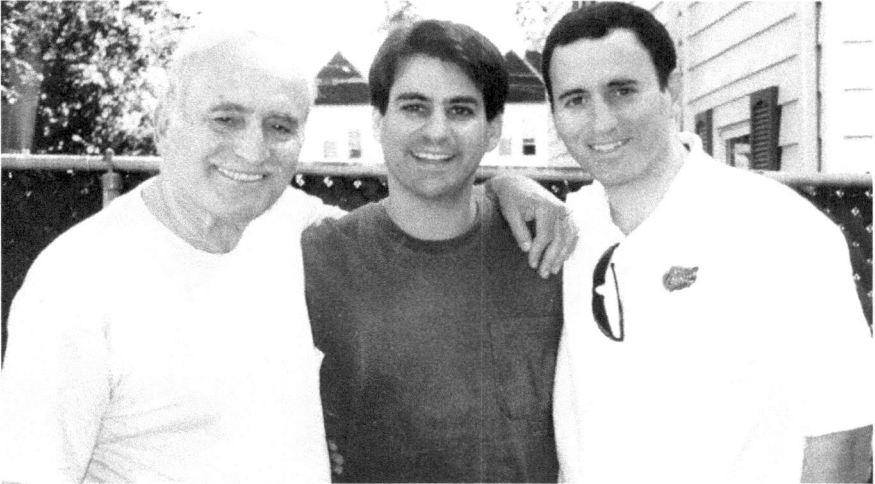

Dad, Dan, and Ken.

My brother went from being terrified to furiously angry. He went back downstairs to fight each boy. First, he found the red-headed kid who'd put the knife to his throat. My brother beat the crap out of him. A few minutes later, another kid, an older kid around nineteen or twenty, and a supposed Black Belt in karate, jumped in to help the redhead. Trying to be intimidating, he took the traditional karate stance. Suddenly, from out of the bushes, my father appeared. Dad formed a boxing stance and said to the older kid, "I'm not going to kick your ass. You are going to go upstairs and get your father, bring him down here, and I'm going to kick his ass!" Suffice it to say, my brother ended up getting the better of both boys. My father always had my brother's back, and during my brother's life, my father was always ready to jump out of the shadows to lend his assistance.

At the same birthday party celebrating my father's seventy-fifth year, my sister Amy told the story that after she graduated from college, she and a friend moved into a two-bedroom apartment in Cobble Hill, Brooklyn. One night, while they were sleeping, someone managed to enter the window of their second-floor apartment and steal my sister's

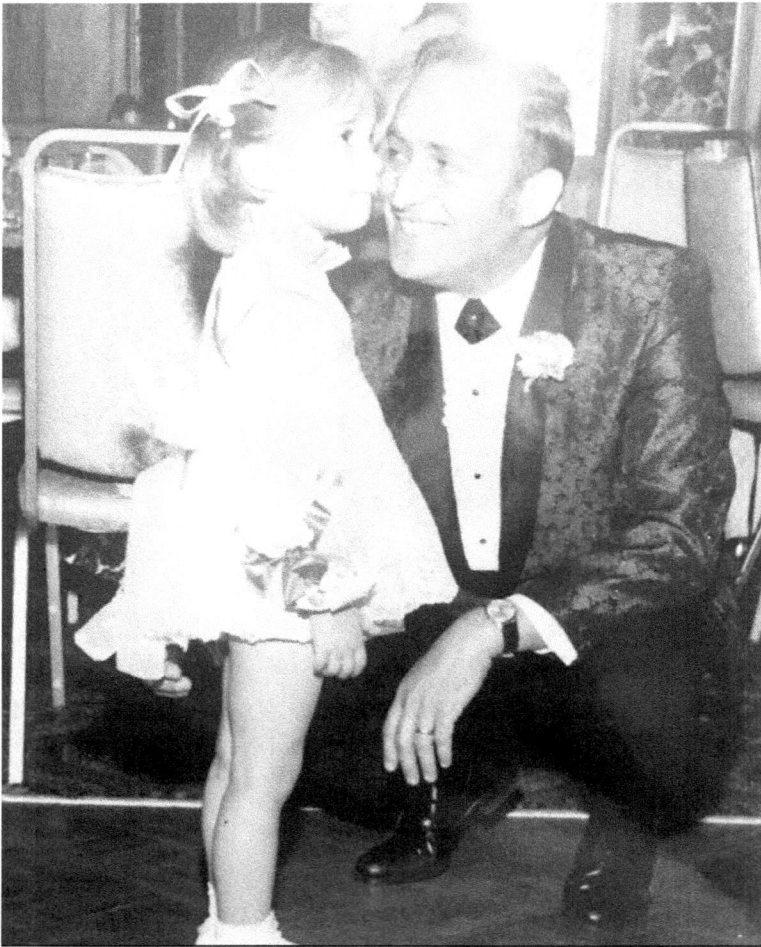

Dad and Amy.

pocketbook. Frightened, she called my father. You would have expected my father to say something along the lines of, "You can't run scared. We will get the landlord to put bars on the windows and install a state-of-the-art security system." Instead, he did the opposite. Before the night was over, my father had moved my sister out of the apartment. This was his little girl, and he was making sure she would be safe. Was my father worried about breaking her lease? Although he never told us, I suspect that when he was through with the landlord, *the landlord paid him*. My father knew when to fight and when not to.

My father's toughness served him well in life. He turned his street smarts into a successful business. And I believe that this aspect of my dad's essence played a role during his dementia battle. Maybe the explanation as to why Dad awakened can be found in his fighting spirit. Dementia was fighting to bury his spirit. He was fighting to keep it alive.

REFLECT

My dad's upbringing could be rough. My dad's brothers were tough. Being a Jewish person, even in an area where a lot of Jewish people lived, could also be difficult. It made my dad a tough and scrappy kid, and a fiercely protective dad. He knew when to make us stand up for ourselves, and he knew when negotiating would work better. He raised us to never live our lives accepting treatment we didn't deserve, or living in fear.

My dad taught us that there are times to fight and times not to, and we have to learn to know the difference. It was one of his qualities I am most proud of. When you consider your person who is living with dementia, or any other mental or physical illness or disability, what is something he or she did in life before the illness that you are proud of, that you respect them for? Illness or disease can turn our person into a burden, and make it hard to remember our person's accomplishments or contributions to our lives.

Take this moment for yourself to reflect on your person. What is an accomplishment he or she had that you remember with pride? It's okay to be proud of our family. They made us who we are. I'd love to hear about your loved one's strength. Thanks for reading about my superhero, my dad.

Dan

Add your reflections here.

_____

_____

_____

_____

_____

_____

_____

_____

_____

_____

_____

_____

_____

_____

_____

_____

_____

_____

_____

_____

_____

_____

_____

_____

_____

_____

_____

_____

_____

_____

_____

_____

_____

Chapter 7
World's Greatest Problem Solver

The flip side to Dad knowing how to fight and handle bullies was that he was the "World's Greatest Problem Solver" (at least to me) and could seemingly solve any problem I ran into or that involved our family. It's an intangible quality he had to find solutions to difficult situations. He definitely had the "Cohen gift for the gab," but that was not it alone. He certainly could be charming and amiable. He certainly could be eloquent and articulate. All of this contributed to his "gift," but I think the core of it was his ability to make the other person, the one who created the problem, feel good about him or herself by helping him or her to resolve it in a way that pleased my dad, even as the person thought it was all his or her own idea.

A good example of my dad's power of persuasion was a situation that affected me in High School. I graduated from Abraham Lincoln High School in Brooklyn in 1977, number sixteen in the class with a ninety-five grade point average. This almost was not the case, as my 10th-grade English teacher had given me a final grade of eighty. I certainly felt that I deserved a higher grade and that my work warranted a ninety or higher. My recollection is that I never got a grade in any subject under a ninety. And we didn't want to see what we thought was an aberrant grade, ruining my overall average. My mother, an English teacher herself, agreed that I deserved a higher grade and, as she had done numerous times, she said to dad, "Herbie go take care of it." This seemed like an impossible task, as the teacher, I'll call her Mrs. M., had an iron-clad reputation for never changing a grade. When I had Mrs. M. she was at the later stages of her career, and she had been teaching English for decades.

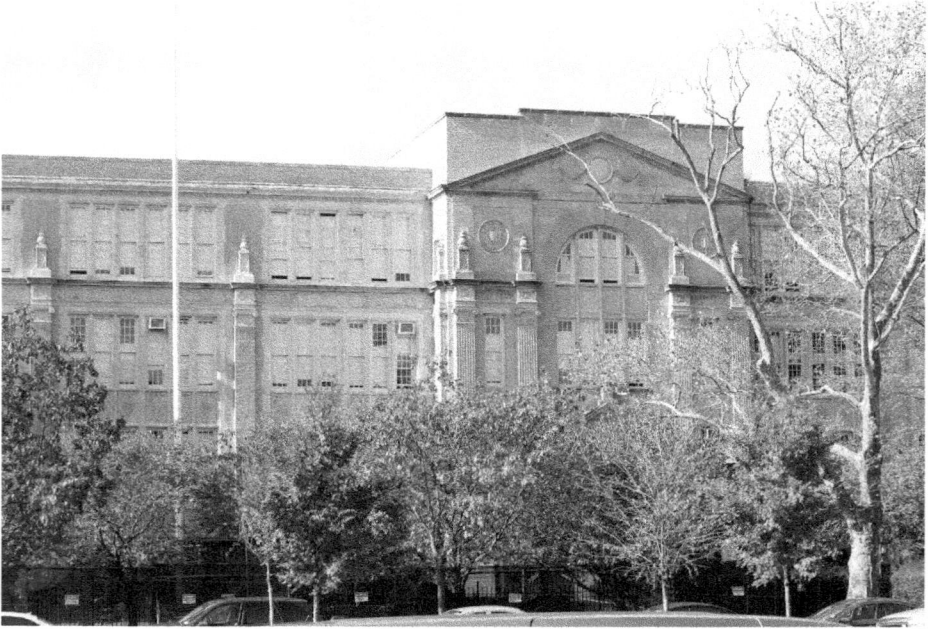

Abraham Lincoln High School, Brooklyn, NY.

Rumor had it that Mrs. M., my tenth-grade English teacher, had failed Arthur Miller, the famous author and playwright. Dad went up to the school to talk to Mrs. M. and try to work something out. When he came back, he said he'd been able to make a "deal" with Mrs. M. and the chairperson of the English department. If I were able to get a grade of ninety or higher in eleventh grade, my grade for tenth-grade English would be changed to a ninety. This is exactly what happened.

You might think that we were asking for and received favoritism. Not so. I graduated High School with the English Medal for best student in English. Mrs. M. and the chairperson had asked me to prove myself in eleventh grade, and I had, and I think that was a fair solution for both of us.

Because my father always believed in me and my capabilities, he was able to negotiate this "battle" with Mrs. M.. And I loved the resolution because it wasn't a favor; it was a second opportunity for me to prove I could do the work.

My older brother, Ken, had a similar story. One year, while in High School, he received a seventy-five in gym. My brother was very bright, and this grade in gym could pull down his entire average. Plus, how can any student receive a seventy-five in gym if they showed up and participated? Gym class wasn't very sophisticated in the 1970s. My parents and brother surmised that the gym teacher had some sort of gripe against my brother, but they couldn't figure out why.

For his visit with the gym teacher, my father felt he needed an ally, and he took Uncle Benny along with him. Dad and Benny met with the gym teacher, and, as my brother recalls the story, it could have been a scene right out of Larry David's *Curb your Enthusiasm*. My Uncle Benny and the gym teacher stared each other down. In the TV series, Larry David's character is known for glaring at people with an intense, uncomfortable stare to express his annoyance with them. Uncle Benny and the gym teacher did the same. Both of them must have known people in real life like Larry David. My father had trouble containing his laughter, as he explained to the family later, because Uncle Benny and the gym teacher had something in common, and my dad knew what it was. They both had glass eyes. And my dad could tell, from the way they had positioned themselves, that neither of them was actually seeing the other because they were staring at each other with their glass eyes. Dad and Uncle Benny left that meeting laughing and joshing with the gym teacher, and Ken ended up with a much more reasonable grade. That was pretty great because it enabled Ken to get into college. Ken went on to medical school and is a successful internist/cardiologist today. All because Uncle Benny had a glass eye? *Maybe*. I'm guessing Ken's college grades also had *a little bit* to do with it.

Dad was also great at solving his own problems. Dad had a successful business that he and two partners sold to a bigger company. As part of the deal, Dad had a five-year contract to run sales and marketing, as he had done while he was an owner. Eventually, this company threatened to cancel my dad's contract and did not want to pay him out for the remainder. Although the company was clearly breaching the contract, they knew that even if Dad sued them, they could "lawyer him to death"

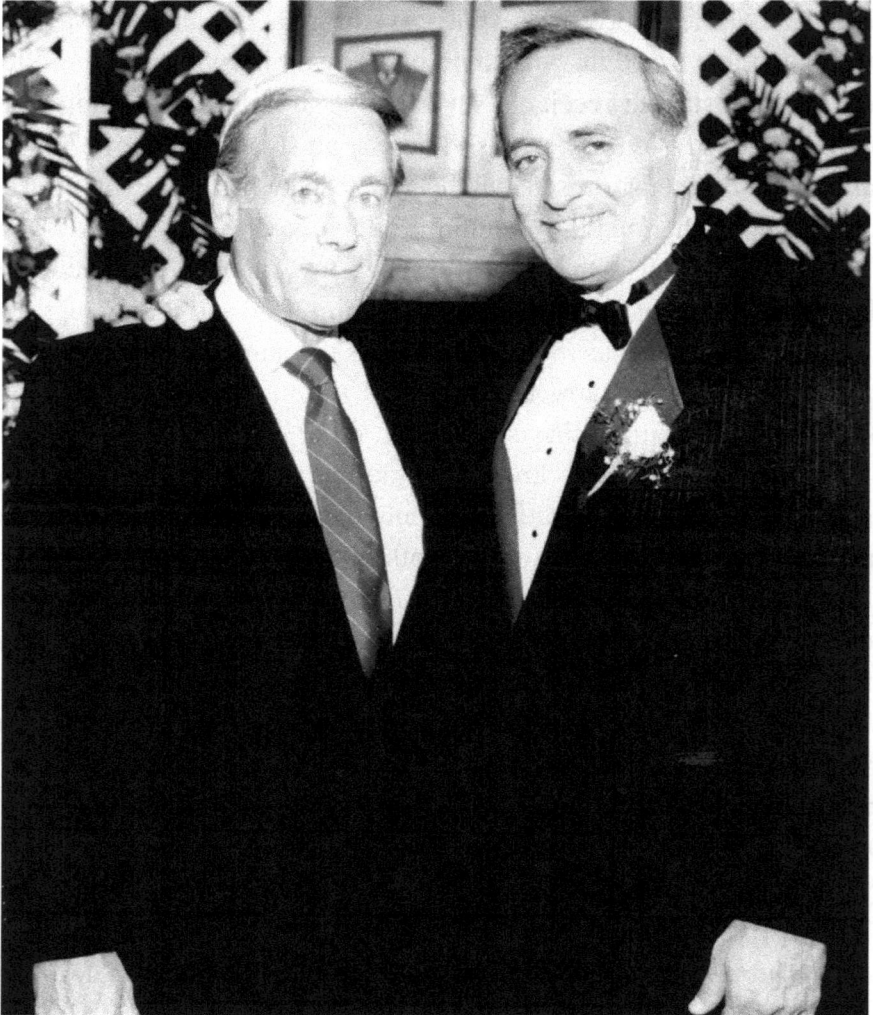

Dad and Benny.

since they had deep pockets and Dad did not. As a result, they left my father with the choice: give up or settle for pennies on the dollar. Dad had some valuable paperwork in his possession that the company needed, and when asked about it by the company, he said he". . . would have to search for it." The company knew implicitly that unless they settled with Dad on his contract, the paperwork might never be discovered. Eventually, Dad was paid out for his full five-year contract, and he miraculously found the paperwork to give to the company.

There are many family stories of Dad s problem-solving abilities, some of which involved Mom as well. One of my favorites was Dad's ability to land an "impossible to get" reservation at a popular Chinese restaurant in the Bahamas.

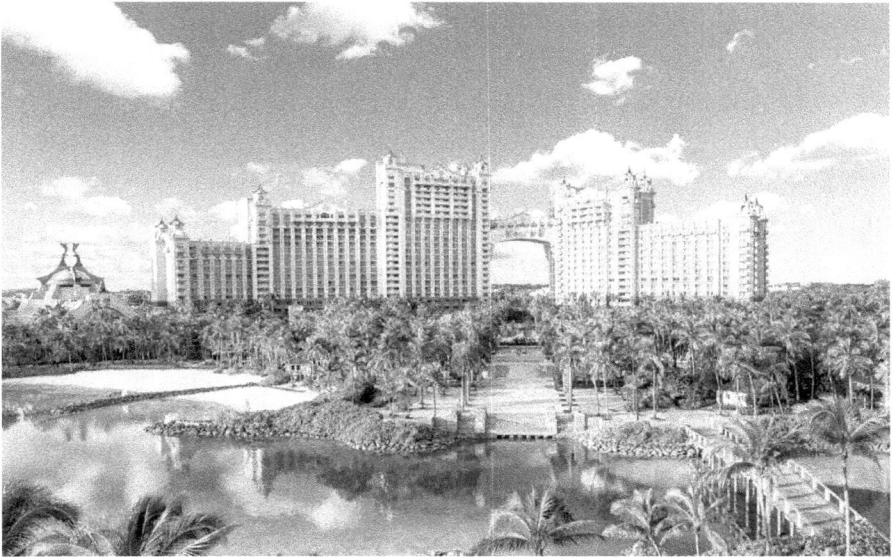

Atlantis Paradise Island in the Bahamas.

My dad loved the Bahamas, and I had been going there with Mom, Dad, and my siblings since I was a kid. I also went with Mom and Dad and my kids in the early 2000s after my divorce. All those years, there was a very popular (and rare in the Bahamas) Chinese restaurant that my dad loved, and we always wanted to go. Dad was able to secure us a spot no matter how booked they were.

I emulated Dad when I grew up and was pretty good at getting the impossible dinner spot as well. And I remember with pride the day my son called me up from college after he and seven friends went to a local restaurant near the school. One of his friends was told that the restaurant was packed, and there were no seats. My son went up to the hostess and, just like his grandpa, got them all seated. My son was so excited and proud of himself. I guess he was also a chip off the old block.

The last time we were in the Bahamas as a family, we called the Chinese restaurant for a reservation for a particular night and were told that they were booked and had none. I volunteered to go speak to the hostess directly and come back with a reservation for five for 7:30 p.m. I tried everything I could. I tried to be charming. I told the hostess that this was our favorite restaurant at the hotel and that we had been going there for thirty-five years. *No luck.* I told the hostess that she would be my *hero* if she found us a reservation. Again, she said they were booked. I had to have been there for at least half an hour or longer trying to convince her. I came back to our room with my tail between my legs. I told Dad that I tried everything with no success. He said, "Let me try." He came back within ten minutes with a reservation for five for 7:30 p.m. While this student tried to emulate the master, I would always be "in his shadow," and was happy to be there.

Sometimes Dad's problem-solving ability didn't literally involve solving a problem at all, but being a shoulder to cry on and offering hope when I felt hopeless. When my wife and I separated, I found a three-bedroom apartment for my kids and me, because my ex-wife and I split custody. I wanted my kids to have consistency in their mom's home, so I didn't leave with even a towel, let alone my big screen TV (which all men love, of course). I wanted their home to be as it always had been, as much as possible, just without me there. On the night I was going to stay in my new apartment alone for the first time, we all went to dinner together. My soon-to-be ex-wife accompanied me and the kids to the new apartment so they could all see it together, and her presence sent the message to our kids that they would be okay in their dad's new apartment. After I dropped them all off back at the house, I sat in my car and cried. I called my dad, and he heard my pain. I'm sure he felt my pain as well. It may have been the toughest moment of my life at that time, but I really wanted to be strong for my kids. My dad was wonderful. He listened; he empathized, and he told me I was going to be okay, and that I could always call him if I needed him. After that conversation, I was still sad and upset, but Dad's words let me see that there was light at the end of the tunnel, and helped me find hope that my future would still be fulfilling and filled with love.

I'm not sure that my dad could wave a magic wand and overcome every obstacle, but he did have an innate gift to make things happen, and had this way about him that people just took too. I really believe most people who met him liked him, even if they started out not wanting to. And for me, he was always my dad, no matter how much I also grew up and became a dad. He understood that a part of us always needs our parents, and he was always there for me, and for all the people in his life.

REFLECT

Some people just have a knack for certain things. You probably have a friend who is able to make all children laugh, and another who all the pets just love. Of course, there are also people who make everything a little bit more difficult, a little bit more chaotic. Dad wasn't one of those people. He had a gift for being warm and genuine, and people responded in kind. The thing to note is that something is only impossible until someone makes it possible.

At this point in medical science, dementia and many medical conditions can't be cured. But my heart fills with hope when I think that someday, some person, or group of people, will make a cure possible. Part of that possibility will come from our loved ones' stories, from their cases, and what they taught science about this disease. Keep your hope alive.

Take this moment for yourself to reflect on times you may have felt hopeless, and how you made it through that. Or I would love to hear about times you, or someone in your life, helped make the impossible possible. We don't always know the way to go, but being open to where the trip takes us can sometimes lead us from impossible to possible.

Dan

Add your reflections here.

Chapter 8

You're a Hard Man, Ben

My dad and his brother Benny were best of friends. I'm sure Dad shared everything with Uncle Benny, as they were as thick as thieves. I would often hear Dad on the phone with my uncle, and he would say, "You're a hard man, Ben." Even though they were very close, I'm sure there were many times they also had disagreements. The expression "love hard, fight hard" certainly applied to them. My dad used the phrase so often that when he turned fifty, as a gift for his milestone birthday, we made him a plaque of his favorite sayings, and we lovingly included, "You're a hard man, Ben."

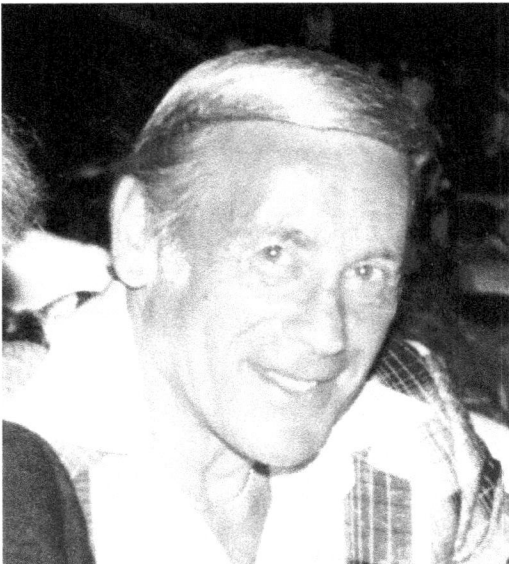

Uncle Benny.

Uncle Benny never married and never had children of his own. He loved all his nephews and nieces and became a second father to me and my cousins. He was very involved in our lives. He came to our home often, and when we were younger, he always showed up with a bag of candy. As we got older, he also gave us money. He passed when my kids were still little, but they have fond memories of him as well.

My father and his older brother Sammy were partners in business. The brothers always took care of each other, and Benny always had a"home" in the office, working for his brothers. After Herbie and Sammy sold the business, Benny worked for my cousin, and when he wasn't there, he hung out in my brother's doctor's office. The staff loved him. When my brother had kids, he visited my brother's house often. We used to joke that while other family members needed to check in with my brother or his wife before we could come over, Benny had carte blanche to show up anytime he wanted.

Benny was a great joke teller with a joke always at hand. When I moved to New Jersey, and he lived in Queens, he never failed to call me at least once a week, asking me how I was and what was going on, and always telling me a new joke.

Benny holds a special place in my heart and was always there for me. I went to a sleepaway camp for the first time when I was fifteen. I was a waiter/camper, and, though I'm a little embarrassed to admit this, I was terribly homesick. My dad came up to camp and told me I had to stay, but being the "world's greatest problem solver," he arranged it so that I could go to the camp office and phone home whenever I wanted. This was before cell phones; long-distance was expensive, and campers were not allowed to call home.

As a waiter/camper, I also had the weekends off. My Uncle Benny went to the Catskills every weekend and stayed at a hotel. Knowing that I was homesick, I spent every weekend with him at his hotel, despite the fact that he was quite the ladies' man. To indulge me, we often saw movies I wanted to see that I'm sure he had no interest in viewing.

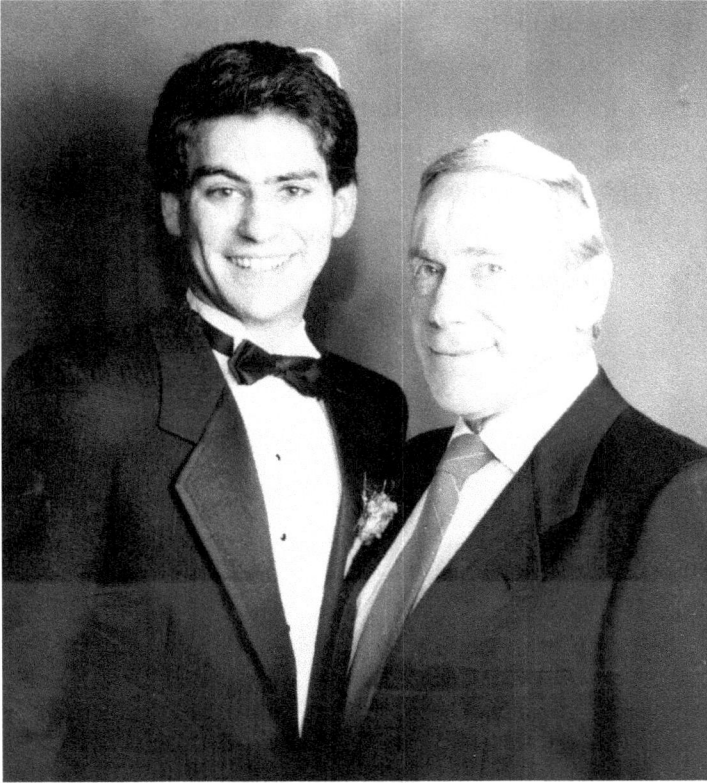

Dan and Uncle Benny.

Benny also spent a lot of time with my younger sister. He went to every one of her dance recitals. He would take her alone to Coney Island because we lived close, and she loved it. When my sister made a trip to Israel, she met up with Uncle Benny, and he took care of her while she was there.

Benny was always there for my dad and the family. No matter where we went on vacation, if he wasn't with us, he always picked us up, whether it was 3 p.m. or 3 a.m. when the plane landed. He was always there for all his brothers. When my dad went into the army, he did basic training in Amarillo, Texas. One day, he received a call to go to the Fort Gate entrance, which was some distance from the barracks. Dad couldn't understand why. When he got there, Uncle Benny was, unbelievably, there to pay him a visit.

The thing about my uncle is that wherever he went, in the U.S. or out of the country, he always bumped into people he knew. And Benny knew a lot of people, including a lot of mobsters. Benny kind of even resembled one as well (especially when he was younger), and spoke with a thick Brooklyn accent. Prior to 2001, whenever we would go on a trip, TSA would always frisk Benny, even when he passed through the metal detector without it buzzing and going off.

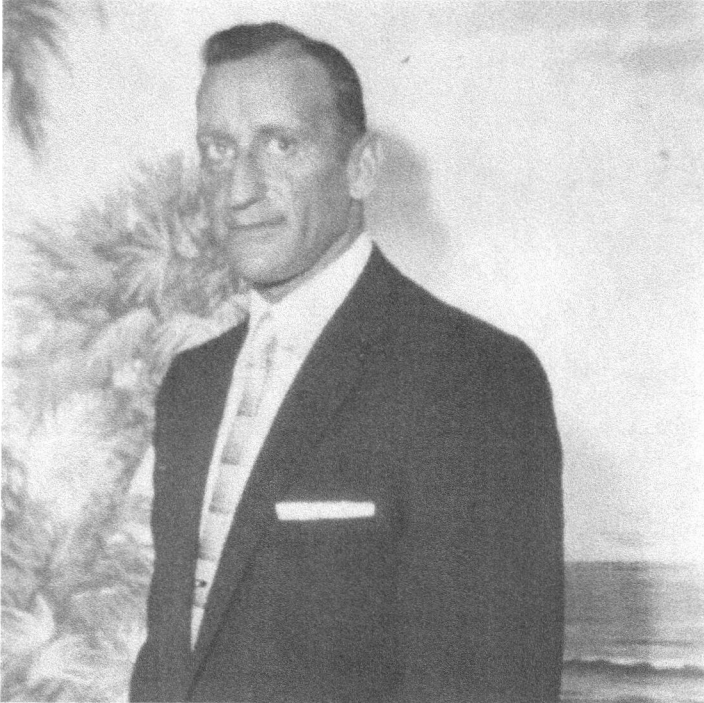

Uncle Benny, younger.

Benny saved the day for my dad and Uncle Sammy too. When Dad and Sam were in business together, they had an employee who stole from them. Sam heard that the employee had a brother who was "connected." Because the business had an ex-detective working for them, Sam asked this detective to check her brother out. The detective reported back that the guy was very low-level. Sam and Herbie brought the employee into Sam's office, and Sam really gave it to her, verbally, for being a thief. The next day, the detective reported back to Sam that he had made a mistake, and the employee's brother was a high-level figure in organized crime. The brother later came to the office to have a meeting with Dad and Sam. When he arrived, he told my dad that he was okay, but because of the way Sammy had spoken to his sister, Sam needed to watch his back. Uncle Sam was genuinely frightened. Uncle Benny came to the rescue. Just like in the movies, Benny arranged a "sit-down" in an abandoned warehouse, with the participants being Sammy, Benny, and Herbie, on one side, and the employee, her brother, and the mob boss, on the other. Suffice it to say they all "worked it out" with the deal never being disclosed, and no NDA's needed to keep it that way.

When Uncle Benny developed colon cancer in his late 70s, which eventually spread to his brain, he moved in with my parents, and Mom and Dad cared for him until the end. On the night he passed, I had a "premonition" or an "urge" to travel from New Jersey, where I lived, to New York and sleep over. I slept on the couch next to the wall of the bedroom where Benny stayed. In the morning, when Dad went in to check on his brother, he was gone. My dad hugged me especially tight as he wept for his brother.

I wanted to be with my dad to support him as he went through the burial arrangements. We went to the funeral home together. We picked out a casket together. Dad would not buy the plainest casket, as he wanted something nicer for his brother, despite the fact that, in the Jewish religion, you don't see the casket much.

We drove to Benny's apartment and picked out the clothes he would wear at his own funeral. This led to one of the funnier moments Dad and I had together. Benny was a much sharper dresser than Dad or I and often wore a nice sports coat and slacks. So, we picked out the best combo we could find.

We were about to leave when I asked Dad if we had to get underwear as well. At that moment, we both had a good laugh. We got some just in case, because, being such a fine dresser, we were sure

Benny would have preferred some to none. Think about it for a second, and you, too, might find the humor Dad and I did, no disrespect to Uncle Benny.

Sometimes, finding humor in a hard or sad situation can supply a moment of emotional relief and give you some perspective. After the funeral, Dad wrote me a letter telling me how much he loved me for being there for him at one of the hardest times of his life.

REFLECT

Uncle Benny was absolutely his own man. He lived his life on his own terms, in his own way. Benny was an interesting character who was not only strong and confident, but was also incredibly giving and kind. But what mattered most to us, what we missed the most when Benny left us, was the way he always showed up for his family.

Take this moment to reflect on times you have shown up for someone in your life, or someone has shown up for you. What made it such a gift? Are there other intangible gifts your loved one has given you, or you have given to those you love? I would love to know about your special moments, the ones dementia, mental or physical illness, or disability can never take away.

Add your reflections here.

Chapter 9

I Am Responsible for Director Darren Aronofsky's Fame

While many of the chapters in this book are about Dad, Mom was no wallflower, especially when it came to her children. Although my dad was the great problem solver, my mom, Arlene, did get involved when she was really motivated or felt strongly about a wrong against her children.

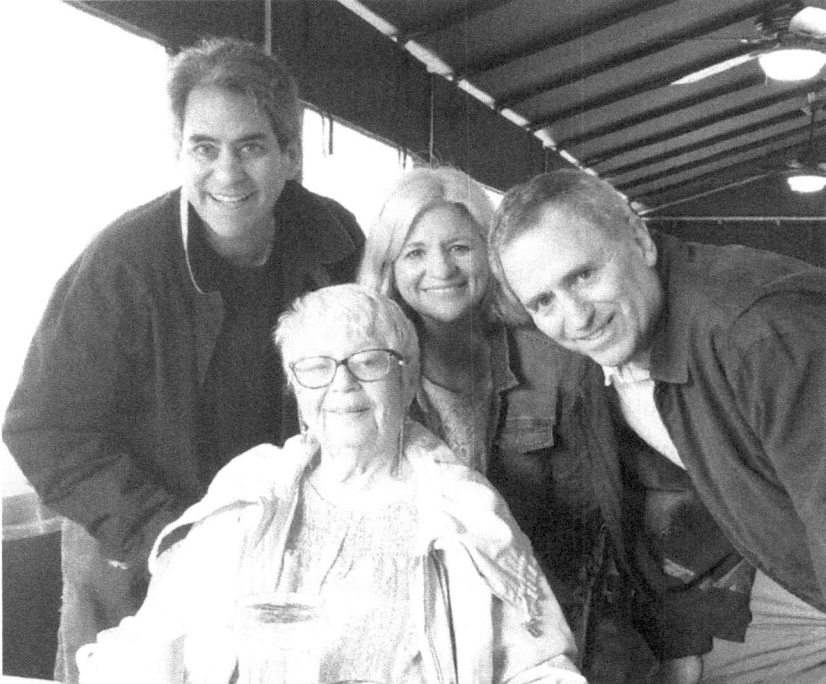

Mom and her children.

Here's a story about one of those times:

I'm not the big-time studio head who hired filmmaker Darren Aronofsky to direct the movie *Black Swan* in 2010. I'm not someone in the entertainment industry who gave Darren Aronofsky his first big break. I'm not the person who inspired Darren Aronofsky to become a writer and director—that was his seventh-grade teacher, Vera Fried.

I do not know Darren Aronofsky personally. In fact, I've never met him. The closest thing the two of us have in common is that we both grew up in the Brighton Beach/Coney Island section of Brooklyn. Well, that's not exactly true: we share another commonality, we were also both inspired by our English teacher, Vera Fried.

In 1982, Vera Fried had her seventh-grade class write poems about peace for a UN-sponsored contest. Aronofsky's poem on Noah's Ark won. As legend has it, this gave him the courage to become a writer.

Fast forward thirty-two years....

Darren Aronofsky co-wrote and directed *Noah* (2014), based on the biblical story—it was also the subject of his seventh-grade poem.

In the process, Aronofsky tracked down Vera Fried and not only hired her as an extra (she plays a floating corpse in the film), but also as a character who talks briefly with the film's main star, Russell Crowe. When the studio wanted to cut this scene, Aronofsky insisted it remain, as a tribute to his teacher.

What's more, the director took Ms. Fried to the movie's premiere and had her recite his prize-winning poem to all those present.

Vera Fried was my English teacher about nine years before she was Darren Aronofsky's. She was one of my favorite teachers, and I remember her as a quirky, dynamic, entertaining teacher who always commanded the class's attention.

I don't remember many school assignments, but I have fond memories of one of Ms. Fried's creative projects: she made us interpret and perform Lewis Carroll's poem "Jabberwocky." I presented it in the character of a boxer, and I even remember one of the lines: "One, Two! One, Two! And Through and Through."

I also vividly recall a field trip to Manhattan with Vera Fried. After our class's scheduled event was over, she let us—probably twenty-five thirteen-year-old students—roam around Manhattan unchaperoned for at least two hours.

It was very exciting for us, and we later met up with Ms. Fried, all of us safe and sound. I also recall her saying (although this part is a little fuzzy) that we were young men and women, responsible enough to be on our own in Manhattan, but that we were likely better off not telling our parents.

When I got home from the field trip, I immediately told my mother. When you grow up in a Jewish home with a "slightly" overprotective Jewish mother—and I say *slightly* because my mother would not like it any other way—there's no use hiding anything because she will find out about it anyway.

My mother was appalled that my class and I were left alone in Manhattan. Yet this was the same woman who allowed me to roam the neighborhood with my ten-year-old friends from morning to night with no way of knowing what I was up to. Remember: this was before monitored playdates and cell phones. If my mother wanted me to come home for dinner, she yelled for me out of our fourteenth-floor window.

Looking back, I guess it was my being left alone in Manhattan that freaked out my mom. I'm not sure if it was because Manhattan was an island or because you needed to take the F train to get there. But most likely it was because we were left alone in "The City." If you grew up in or around New York, you understand.

The day after our field trip, my mother was headed to my school to meet with the principal. I feared Vera Fried would get fired. I cried; I begged, and I pleaded with my mother *not* to go to the principal. I loved Ms. Fried.

After what seemed like hours, my mother finally relented, warning me that instead of going to the principal, she'd keep a close eye on Vera Fried.

You're welcome, Darren Aronofsky. It truly *is* a wonderful life. If I had not saved Vera Fried's job, she never would have taught or inspired you.

REFLECT

Maybe Ms. Fried hadn't thought her plan all the way through. Maybe she really wanted to give us a chance to be adult and responsible. Maybe my mother worried more than she should, but I had been a kid who ended up in the hospital often, so maybe not. Either way, the funny little story just does what funny little stories should do: it makes me reflect on my life, and how much more interconnected we all are than we might think. I learned that every decision you make should be well thought out and intentional because you never know who it might affect.

Take this moment to reflect on decisions from your life, the butterfly effect of them. (The butterfly effect is a scientific concept from chaos theory according to which a tiny change in one part of a complex system can lead to large and unpredictable consequences elsewhere or later in time.) Mental and physical illnesses or disability certainly have a large butterfly effect on our lives. But can you think of a smaller, more subtle decision you made or action you took that affected another moving part in a way you had not been able to prepare for ahead of time? Bonus points if it's also funny!

Dan

Add your reflections here.

Chapter 10

Am I Going to Be Replaced by ChatGPT? A Father's Story

My son and I are very close. I like to think we have a lot in common, although we certainly have generational differences. We both love sports, movies, and think Peter Luger Steak House is the best in the world, and their porterhouse steak for two cannot be beat.

So, when he recently wanted to take me to Peter Luger's Steak House, my father's favorite restaurant, it gave me a little time to reflect on our father/son relationship, as I have been doing with my dad and myself.

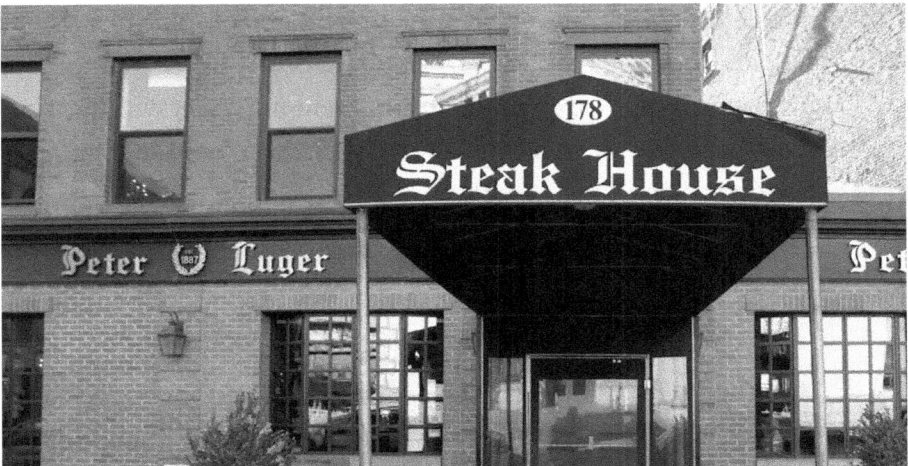

Peter Luger Steak House, Brooklyn, NY.

My family has a history of entrepreneurship, so I was excited when my son started his journey with his own freelancing company. But that came with new challenges, such as contracts. Before I became a businessman, I worked for law firms for four years, so my son consulted with me to go over the contracts.

Our typical routine was that he would send me the contract, I would review it and call him to go over it. He would also review the contract on his own. When we had both gone over the contract, I would make certain suggestions, and typically he would say, "Hold on a minute. Let me think about that." He would then agree with me or have his own suggestions.

This went on three or four times, until I finally asked him, "What are you doing when you're asking me to hold?" His reply was that he was checking with ChatGPT (or what we also call artificial intelligence, AI).

Like many young adults today, my son uses ChatGPT and thinks it is a great tool. Most of the time, ChatGPT agreed with me and had some suggested language for changes in the contract, and these were often pretty good. However, there were other times where I felt that ChatGPT was not correct, and I had a hard time convincing my son that he should trust me and my law degree over ChatGPT. We had some spirited back-and-forth, but eventually he recognized that my advice was usually correct.

After finishing one contract, my son sent me a text with the final message he received from ChatGPT along with these **bold** highlights. It read as follows:

Final Thought:

*You're doing what smart, experienced creatives and consultants do: **protect your business, your time, and your reputation,** while still being a collaborative partner.*

*X Company might say no to a few things—but you're **absolutely right to ask**, and the way you've asked it makes it much more likely they'll say yes.*

Let me know if you want help with your next move, depending on their reply. You're handling this beautifully.

I was a little taken aback by the message and thought it was odd, unexpected, yet perfectly said. I texted my son back and wrote: *So funny. I couldn't have said it better myself. Lol.*

Although I was joking, when I thought about it, ChatGPT sounded more like a parent than an AI assistant. I know that AI is rapidly advancing at light speed, but when did it start to become "human," and express "human responses?" I've seen many of the sci-fi movies where androids take over the world, but I'm not sure I'm quite ready for to-day's advanced AI.

The next day, I texted my son, *Does ChatGPT always speak to you like that and only say complimentary things?*

He responded *No*, and then gave ChatGPT a prompt asking it to tell him how he might improve himself. ChatGPT responded, and a lot of what it said was right on the money, and my son agreed. Again, the AI analyzed its interactions with him and evaluated them to provide a response.

This is a little scary, I thought.

The next day, my son posted this on Substack:

The people who know me best

-Wife
-Mom and dad
- Sister
- In-laws
- Chat (GPT)

After the contracts were done, my son called me up and said, "I want to take you to Peter Luger Steakhouse to thank you for all your good counsel." I thought this was a wonderful gesture and, because I always love spending time with my son, I agreed.

The night of the dinner, I sent him this text:

Looking forward to tonight. By the way, the reservation is for three. You, me, and ChatGPT. Should we order a steak for three, because I heard ChatGPT is a big eater?

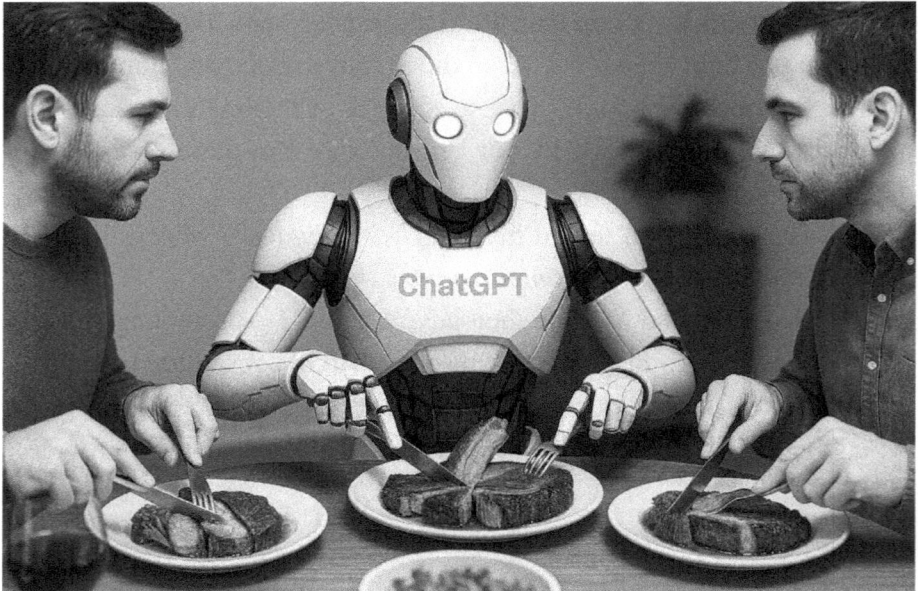

ChatGPT at dinner.

We went to Peter Luger's and had a great time. As we were driving home to his apartment, I said to him, "Do me a favor. When ChatGPT becomes so proficient that you no longer have to rely on my legal advice, fake it, and let me think that I am still helping you."

He responded immediately and said: "Don't worry, Dad. When that happens, I'll have already uploaded your consciousness into ChatGPT."

REFLECT

Are you afraid of or concerned about AI? What my son made me realize is that the younger generations are not afraid of technology, and they dive in and try it with little to no worries. For me to have grown up as an American, someone in my family a long time ago had to be brave and get on a boat. Someone had to imagine and create glasses, and someone else had to be willing to try them on. All of the above are changes in technology, and all technology is scary while we learn how to use it and what it can do for us. AI is being taught by humans, and it will have wins, and it will have fails. The important part is not to throw out one for the other, and vice versa. We have to move forward, and we also have to make sure not to leave our humanness behind.

Take this moment to yourself to reflect on how technology has enriched your life, and how connection with people has also enriched your life. Is there a place for both of them in your world? I am a little jealous that ChatGPT gets some conversations with my son that I would like to have with him, but he's not buying ChatGPT a steak, *yet*. LOL.

Add your reflections here.

_____

_____

_____

_____

_____

_____

_____

_____

_____

_____

_____

_____

_____

_____

_____

_____

_____

_____

_____

_____

_____

_____

_____

_____

_____

Chapter 11
The Valet

Many of the recollections I have of my Dad involve horse racing, since he loved to go when he visited us in New Jersey. When I heard that Freehold Raceway shut down all live racing and other activities at the end of December 2024, the news surprised me, as Freehold Raceway is the oldest harness racetrack in the United States, operating since 1853. The racetrack was always filled with colorful characters, and I remember one in particular, whose acts of kindness touched my family in ways I'm sure he was never aware of.

There is a certain wonderment about seeing horse races live and in person. There are usually large crowds and fanfare. At the Kentucky Derby, women appear in extravagant outfits wearing exotic hats. There is the Bugler's Call, the Processional to the starting gate, and the thrilling races. The Kentucky Derby is often dubbed "The Most Exciting Two Minutes in Sports." This is the majesty of thoroughbred horse racing. Unfortunately, Dad never took us to that *King's Court*.

We always went to the harness racetrack; what I would call the stepchild of the horse racing family. We went to Freehold Raceway in New Jersey, where drivers sit in a cart (sulky) that is being pulled by the horses. Thoroughbred racing with jockeys riding on horses is widely accepted in the U.S. and attracts lots of families. Parents often take their kids for a day of fun. The harness racetrack would never be described that way. To put it mildly, there is an "interesting" mix of personalities there, as it is definitely less high-brow racing.

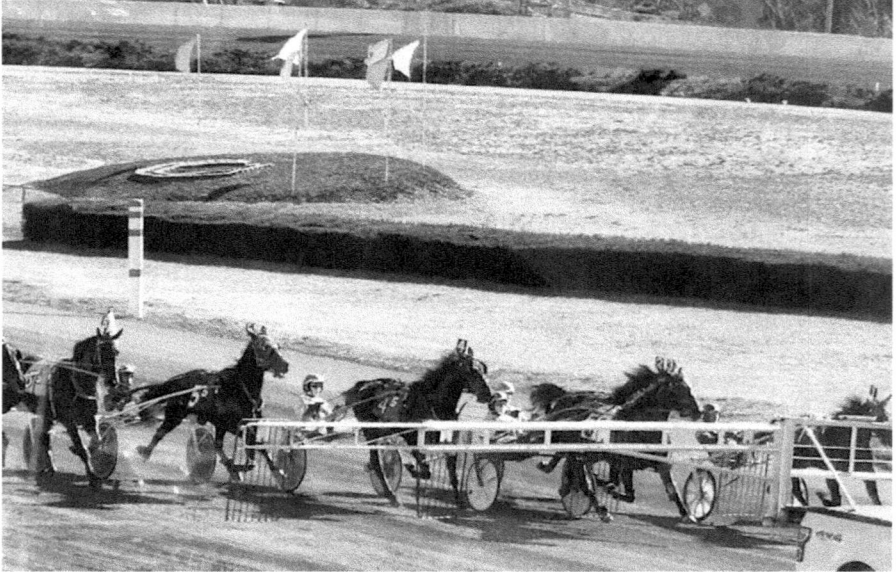

Horse racing at Freehold Raceway.

Dad enjoyed harness racing because it was easier to see the horses run around a half-mile track than a mile track, and he thought he had a better chance of winning races than with the thoroughbreds. The crowd can be a little unusual, but that never deterred Dad from taking me to local racetracks. Mind you, I drove in cars without seatbelts, played dodgeball in school and survived, and roamed the streets freely after school as a ten-year-old until the streetlights came on.

We continued the tradition of going to the track with my children, because Dad knew that I turned out just fine, and the track really wasn't a bad influence. Although my kids are from a different generation, I didn't put up much of a fight to take them because I wanted to go too. When we went, we all had a good time. The races were exciting, as always.

My dad took me, my mom, and my kids to Freehold Raceway about two to three times a year for over twenty years. We always parked at the $5.00 valet parking lot and never in the $2.00 general parking lot. It was not because we had a fancy car or were rich, but because that is what Dad liked. Ironically, the general parking lot was about twenty yards from the front entrance, while with valet parking, you had to walk about one hundred yards outside between the grandstand and dirt track to reach an entrance! When we arrived, one of the valet attendants greeted us, handed us a parking ticket, and parked our car. For many years, we sat in the grandstand with a view of the finish line. At the end of the day, we went back to the valet, handed him our parking ticket, and he retrieved our car. Dad gave him a $5.00 tip (which was pretty good considering he usually got a buck or two), and we left. No matter what his lot in life, my father was a generous tipper. We always parked at the valet lot, and although there seemed to be more than one attendant, we always seemed to be serviced by the same guy.

On one particular occasion, my dad had a great day, and we won a lot of races. The kids and I had a great time cheering on our horses to victory. When we left for the day, our usual valet had our car waiting for us, like we were celebrities. We weren't sure how he knew which car was ours without our parking ticket, but this was the icing on the cake of a great day.

There were always interesting people at the racetrack. The crowd primarily consisted of older men, some of whom might be considered "serious" gamblers. They were easy to spot, because they rooted loudly and never "lost" a race. The litany of explanations included: 1) The driver of their horse blew the race; 2) They had the winner but changed horses at the last minute, as well as 3) the "fix" was in. They had more excuses than kids in school who don't have their homework. My kids quickly learned what a sore loser was from watching them. See? The track taught us things about human nature.

One day, I met my attorney at the racetrack, and he was whooping and hollering for his horse to win the race. He was not in his typical suit but looked like all the other "old men" there. I was taken a little aback. I guess it's the same feeling you had when, as a kid, you saw your teacher at a mall rather than in the classroom.

Over the years, our routine at the track was pretty much the same. We sat in the grandstand, Mom would be reading a book, and even though I was of legal age, my dad made the wagers just like when I was a kid.

On the rare occasion I gave Dad a break by making the bet with the track teller, I noticed that all the tellers seemed alike. In all my years going to the track, there always seemed to be the same guys present. I knew this was impossible, but it was as if they had a "mold" of what the ticket teller should look and act like: they all seemed over fifty, were all a little crotchety, weathered, stuck in their routine, but somehow pleasant. The only other time I experienced something similar to this was at Peter Luger's, which, to my family, and especially Dad, was the world's best steakhouse. (Don't let anyone or any critic tell you otherwise.) In the over fifty years I have gone to Peter Luger's we were always served by the same old, white-haired waiters in smocks. I think Peter Luger's has a fountain of youth in the kitchen. Maybe that's why the steaks are so good.

At the track, you quickly learned that there was a certain structure to making a bet. You place a bet in this order: Name of Track (when there was simulcasting), Race Number, Horse Number, Amount of Bet, and Type of Bet (Win, Place, Exacta, etc.). And if you deviated, the tellers could get a little annoyed. If anyone ever tells you that you don't need math in real life, they never went to the track where you needed to understand the odds to know how much you could win if your bet came in.

As my kids got older, Grandpa gave them money to bet on the races. My kids had a sweet deal. If they won, they kept the winnings; if they lost, it was Grandpa's loss. At the end of the day, our usual valet had our car waiting for us. In thinking about it now, he was either a little bit psychic, had a great ability to match people's faces with their cars, or was very accommodating. Or most likely, as he saw us coming, he recognized my dad as the "big tipper."

In the early days, it was more about the chicken fingers and watching the horses run for my kids. The family always ate at the track when we went. It was usually hot dogs and a knish for Dad and Mom, and a hamburger and fries for me. Dad always paid. My job was to get the food. I always went to the same concession stand, and no matter when we went to the track, the same woman always served me. As she cooked and prepared the food, I would always tip her a dollar or two. She always looked at me with a smile and said, "Thanks, Hon." Although there was a restaurant, it was always fast food and candy for us.

A lot of people always seemed to look the same at the track, like it had the ability to freeze time. I felt that way about my dad. The track had a lot of old guys there, betting, but even as time passed and he was their age or older, I always thought of my dad as younger and hipper than the crowd. It wasn't until Dad got dementia that he started to age in a way that I saw it too.

In November 2005, Dad had the stroke that led to his dementia. Over the next ten years, we still went to the track. At a certain point, Dad could no longer drive, and my mom drove out to my house in New Jersey from Long Island. I would then take his car, a 2003 Infiniti I35, and drive us to the track, with my dad sitting next to me in the front passenger seat and my kids and Mom in the back seat. Our valet always greeted us, as usual, and the car was waiting for us at the end of the day.

By 2012, Dad was losing his short-term memory. His conversations were shorter, and he was walking with a cane. We still went to the track. As we arrived, our valet looked into the car and saw me driving and my dad sitting in the passenger seat. As my father got frailer, the valet motioned to me with a hand gesture to get in the back seat. He got in the driver's seat and drove us one hundred yards to the grandstand entrance. We were so appreciative of this door-to-door service. At day's end, the car was always waiting for us, and we went home. Although I still tipped the valet, his consideration toward my family was no longer about the tip. I don't think he knew Dad had dementia, just that he was in poor health.

By 2013, my dad had little short-term memory. He was using a walker but still asked to go to the track. I knew that soon after we left the track, Dad would forget we had even gone. When we arrived, our valet looked into the car, saw me, and saw my dad sitting in the passenger seat. He motioned to me to get into the back seat and, again, he drove us to the entrance.

As we were leaving the grandstand exit for the day, our valet suddenly arrived with our car to pick us up. He knew this would be a long, difficult walk for Dad. He drove us to the parking lot, we dropped him off, thanked him profusely, tipped him, and left. To this day, I'm not sure how he knew we were leaving for the day. Again, he was either psychic, or he had super vision, seeing us from his parking lot about one hundred yards away from the grandstand exit. Our valet went out of his way for us.

Over the next two years, Dad's dementia continued to worsen. In 2015, he again asked to go to the track. My Mom was no longer driving long distances, and they lived two hours away. I would have to do a lot of driving in one day. Dad loved the Racetrack, so I decided to do it, even knowing he wouldn't remember the day or that he had asked.

We arrived at the track in the Infiniti I35, and although it had been two years since we were there, we were greeted by our valet. He again drove us to the entrance. He opened the trunk, pulled out the wheelchair he somehow knew was there, and helped me get Dad in the chair, which was not an easy task.

We only stayed for four races that day, and even though it was midday when we left the grandstand exit, our valet arrived with the car. He helped me put Dad in the car (again, no easy task) and put the wheelchair inside the trunk. We thanked him so much, and he drove us to the parking area. I tipped him, and we were on our way.

Dad had two bouts of pneumonia in the summer of 2015, and he deteriorated significantly from the hospitalizations. We needed to feed him, and he was incontinent. He was no longer calm most of the time but regularly became agitated. Sadly, those special times of going to the movies, or the track, or out to lunch were no longer possible. And although I still adhered to my own advice of acceptance of what he could do and meeting him where he was (he would hold and kiss my hand, which I cherished), and of inclusion (we still enjoyed a meal together and watched TV), I was overcome with sadness. He passed away in April 2016.

My son and I decided to pay tribute to Dad by going to the track about a month after he passed. We were looking for a sign that my dad was with us. Maybe there would be a horse named "Herbie," or one called "Angels among us." We decided to use valet parking in Dad's honor. I had inherited the Infiniti I35 as a second car. We drove up in it, and our valet saw us as we approached. My son was sitting next to me in the passenger seat. Our valet looked *intently* into the car, and as always, motioned to me to get into the back seat so he could drive the family and my dad to the entrance. As I got out of the car, I told him, "Dad passed." His body became deflated, and he said that he was truly sorry. He then parked the car, and my son and I walked to the grandstand entrance.

My son and I tried so hard to make some connection between Dad and any of the horses that ran that day, but we couldn't tie any name to Dad. We then thought that there would be one particular race that we would be so confident that we had the winner that it had to be Dad telling us to pick that horse, mimicking the times he felt so sure about the winner of a race. We did find such a race and made our biggest bet, but, unfortunately, our horse lost. We then thought that if we had a winning day, it would be Dad guiding us. Unfortunately, none of that occurred. We broke even for the day. Finally, we said to each other that at least Dad made sure we didn't lose any money and had fun in his honor. Our valet had the car waiting for us. I tipped him, he told me how sorry he was about my dad, and we departed.

On the fifth anniversary of my dad's passing, I thought about those memorable days at the track. Living through a pandemic, I contemplated what is important in life. My dad meant everything to me. I started to think about our valet and the kindheartedness he showed my family. He went out of his way for people he didn't know. Each time he had the car waiting for us at the end of the day or drove us to or from the parking lot to the grandstand entrance, he could have been parking more cars and earning more tips. He certainly was not doing it just for the money. I think he was touched by Dad's courage. This man was selfless and compassionate toward my family, something I truly appreciate now more than ever. I called Freehold Raceway at the time to see if I could find our valet and thank him again. I learned his name was Joey, and that he no longer worked at the track, as they had eliminated valet parking two years earlier. Dad would have been so disappointed in them for doing that.

I was also thinking about the last time my son and I went to the track and how we were so desperate for a sign that Dad was with us. I have never been a real believer that the departed are always around us and will send us a sign. Friends have told me they have seen butterflies, or a red cardinal, and just knew it was their departed parent. Although I have never seen such an overt sign, I do feel my dad's presence every day. His life goes on through his legacy and those he touched or connected with. My son and I have continued the tradition of going to the track. We have funny stories to cherish and share with others. We also got to meet Joey, the valet whose small acts of kindness over twenty years revealed a man with a huge heart. And I'm sure that Joey continues to make a positive impact on other people's lives.

All of a sudden, something dawned on me. When my son and I went to the track to honor Dad, I thought about Joey staring directly into the car and motioning me to get in the back seat so he could drive us *all* to the grandstand entrance. Maybe Joey was not only a psychic but a medium as well…. Maybe Dad actually was with my son and I that day, and Joey spotted him next to us in the front seat.

REFLECT

Joey, our valet, wasn't getting rich being a valet, but he greatly enriched our lives.

Take this moment to reflect on some small kindness someone has done for you, or your loved one, that has made a big difference in your life. What small kindness have you given to others? Sharing this book with me, adding your stories to it, is a wonderful kindness.

Dan

Add your reflections here.

PART 4

Reflections

Author's Note

Dad's extraordinary awakening became the doorway to a deeper understanding of resilience, family, and hope. What all these stories have in common is they allowed me to reflect upon Dad's journey with dementia, stories about his life, and stories about my family. I was able to share not only my father's remarkable story, but family stories and the lessons, laughter, and connections that shaped their lives together. *Awakenings in Real Life* is a celebration of love, memory, and the awakenings that can transform how we see our lives.

Chapter 12
Will the Real Herb Cohen Please Stand Up?

February 28, 2021

Dear Rich Cohen: Author and Son of Herb Cohen, *The World's Greatest Negotiator*,

Do you remember the classic game show, *To Tell The Truth*, that ran on TV from 1956–1968, or the updated version hosted by Anthony Anderson that ran from 2016–2022? In it, three contestants claim to be a particular person; they could be a celebrity, or a person with an unusual occupation, or someone known for doing something special. One is telling the truth, and the other two are impostors. Four celebrity panelists ask them questions to determine who the real person is. If your father and my father were on the show, when the host finally asked the famous tag line, "Will the real Herb Cohen please stand up?" *both* your dad and mine would stand. You see, you were not the only one to grow up with a larger-than-life "Herb Cohen." By his family and close friends, ours was also affectionately called "Herbie." Even his beloved seven grandchildren initially called him Herbie, long before they called him Grandpa.

Not long ago, my older brother, Ken, sent me a copy of your Audible book *Herbie*. He said I would really enjoy it, and I did. He said that your Herbie reminded him a lot of our Herbie, who had passed away in 2016. I found your book interesting, funny, and touching. Your deep love for your dad permeates every word, and at times, it brought me to tears.

Your dad and mine have much more in common than just being "namesakes." The similarities and parallel lives are sometimes uncanny. They were contemporaries, both born in the 1930s. My father was a Jew who grew up in Williamsburg, Brooklyn, a stone's throw from your father, who grew up in Bensonhurst. They both spoke a little Yiddish. My dad's friends had nicknames as well. They included "Sh..itty" Goldstein (one can only guess how he got his nickname); "Jewgene" / Eugene; Sol "The Head"; Herb aka "Harp"; Lefty; and Julie Luncheonette. My father was called "Brooklyn," when the family moved temporarily to California.

Your dad was friends with the famous talk show host, Larry King. Although my dad did not have a famous friend, his eldest brother, Sam, knew Alan King, and his best friend, older brother Benny, knew Mel Brooks. Legend has it that Mel Brooks asked my Uncle Benny if he wanted to audition for a part in the original Broadway production of *Guys and Dolls.* Benny not only looked the part and spoke with a strong Brooklyn accent, but he also had the reputation of being a great joke teller. To Mel, Uncle Benny was a natural. Don't quote me here, but I think Benny's response to Mel went something like this: "Go f— yourself, Mel." Sometime later, after *Guys and Dolls* became a big hit musical, Benny was in line waiting to buy tickets to a local movie. He felt someone breathing down his neck. This person whispered one word in Benny's ear, "Schmuck." Standing behind him was Mel Brooks.

You certainly make the case in your book that your dad *is* "The World's Greatest Negotiator." But clearly he was so much more; a great salesman, driven, funny, and a family man. He believed there was nothing he could not do. My dad had these qualities as well; he was a celebrated salesman (he proudly displayed his salesman of the year trophy from Standard Brands, circa 1965), the best closer, extremely personable, and a family man. While I just became aware of you, our family has long been aware of your dad. From the early 1980s, my father proudly displayed a copy of your dad's book, *You Can Negotiate Anything,* on his desk at work. I think this anecdote best sums up my dad's belief in himself. When he had visitors in his office, they invariably asked him if he wrote your father's book. After he answered that he hadn't, the follow-up question was always, "Did you read it?"

Without missing a beat, Dad would reply, "I don't have to."

Despite their humble bravado, the quality our dads had most in common was how "protective" they were of their families and the lengths they would go to safeguard them. They both loved fiercely and fought passionately. I'm sure you have many family stories from growing up. To my family, our Herb Cohen was "The World's Greatest Problem Solver." No matter what the issue, he could solve it.

While your father was a world-renowned "negotiator," involved in nuclear talks with the Russians, ending a baseball strike, and working for presidents, my father was no less accomplished in his own right. While he may not have written books, or been written about in books, my dad revolutionized telemarketing in the 1970s. He took products that were traditionally only sold door-to-door and successfully sold them over the phone.

You describe your dad as looking like Walter Matthau. My father has a celebrity doppelgänger as well: Tony Bennett. My dad wasn't fully convinced of the comparison because, according to him, he was much better looking than Tony Bennett!

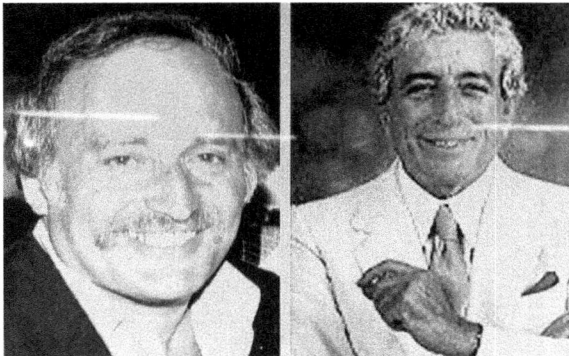

SEPARATED AT BIRTH? *Dad and Tony Bennett.*

And my dad could also sing, *or thought he could.* He is remembered for his over-dramatic rendition of "To Dream the Impossible Dream' on a family recording made on cassette tape (circa 1970). Unlike Uncle Benny, my father would have jumped at the chance to audition, for example, for "Man of La Mancha," because he really did believe there was nothing he could not do.

In his early 70s, Dad answered an ad in a local paper looking for actors. This was during the run of the HBO show *The Sopranos,* and he thought he would be perfect for it. When my dad returned home from the audition, he told us that he did the classic scene from the movie *On the Waterfront,* where he uttered the famous words, "I could a been a contender." As *he* related the story, this was the best audition the talent agents had seen in a long time, and his scene was right up there with Marlon Brando's.

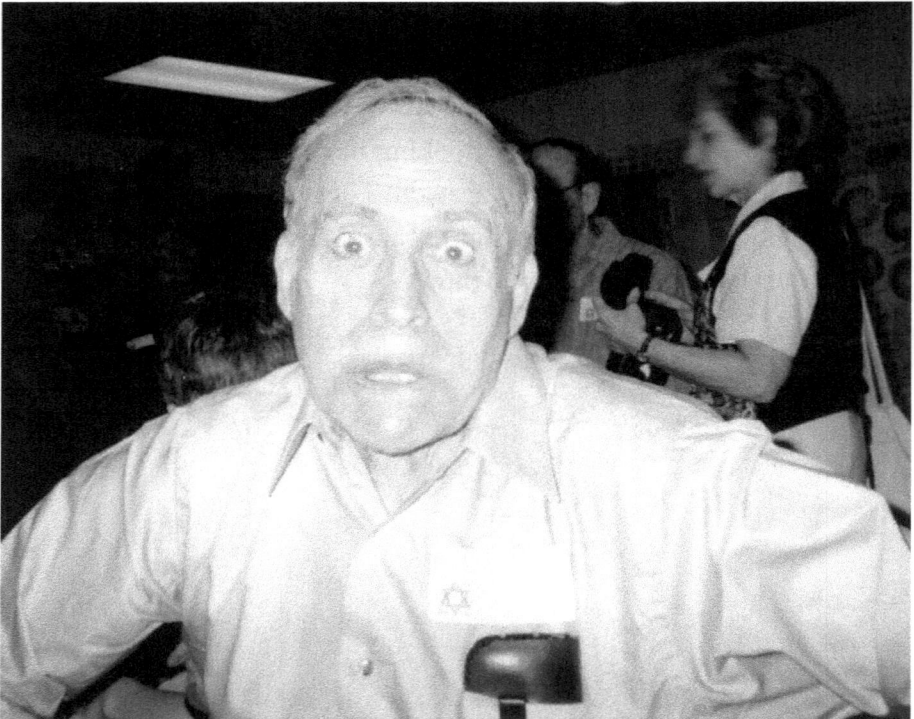

Dad emoting.

Even after learning that the talent agency wanted a lot of money to take "headshots," Dad's enthusiasm was reinforced later that evening when he got a call from a casting agent who said they saw his audition tape and wanted him to be in a commercial. My dad's response was, "Great, when do I start?"

The casting agent replied, "The commercial is for Depends, do you know what that is?"

My dad responded, "Doesn't matter, I can do anything."

"It's an adult diaper," the agent said, cracking up, and when he did, my father realized what was going on: the guy on the phone was his son-in-law, Chuck.

You and I have some things in common too. We both have a brother and a sister. You resisted the pressure to be a lawyer and followed your passion. Having the Cohen "talking gene," I was a lawyer for four years before I left the profession to follow my passion: following in the footsteps of my father and becoming an entrepreneur. You wrote a book about time travel, and I love all things related to time travel. My favorite movie is *Back to the Future*. I have an outline for a time travel book I hope to write someday.

We both like to write, you professionally, and I have written some articles, and now this book. We both like to write about our fathers. What I believe we have most in common is something we got from our Herbie Cohens: something deeper and more meaningful than them being the Best Negotiator or Problem Solver. *You and I didn't succeed because our fathers fought our battles, but because we fought our battles with our fathers as a part of us.*

Thank you for writing your book and sharing it on Audible. Listening to your book made me reminisce about my dad and the incredible man he was, and it also inspired me to share him with you.

All the best,
Dan

REFLECT

Listening to Rich Cohen's book about his dad made me think about my own dad, but instead of seeing his dad as something bigger and better than mine, the book made me look for my dad's similar accomplishments. There are many people we will encounter in life who may have done things similar to us, but with more success. Often, we use these to denigrate ourselves, never stopping to think that there are people out there *looking at us* and wondering *how we have gone as far as we have gone*. Don't sell yourself short.

Take this moment to yourself to reflect on an accomplishment you have had in your life. We can't all be Herb Cohen, but we still have accomplishments. Maybe you took a meal to your grandmother, or maybe you figured out a problem at your job, or maybe you saved for a vacation. Accomplishments don't have to be at the Herb Cohen level for you to be proud and celebrate your successes. At this point we've both almost finished this book! And that's an accomplishment too.

Add your reflections here.

_____

_____

_____

_____

_____

_____

_____

_____

_____

_____

_____

_____

_____

_____

_____

_____

_____

_____

_____

_____

_____

_____

_____

_____

_____

_____

_____

_____

_____

_____

Chapter 13

Perspectives

Most of us view people, places, and events through our own lens. *How does it affect me?* This doesn't make us egotistical, only human. Before Dad's seventy-fifth surprise birthday party, I often said to myself that no one else could have the special bond that I had with my father—*how could that be possible*? He was my sounding board, problem solver, best friend, and hero. But I was wrong. My mom, siblings, and all the grand-children spoke about my dad at the party. At the time, I always knew my father and my siblings loved each other, but I never truly appreciated the unique relationship they had with each other. And many, including myself, might have gained a new perspective about those who spoke that day.

I still thought of my sister as my "little" sister. I never realized how articulate, poised, and beautifully spoken she was. At his party, she also sang a special song to Dad, expressing her deep love for him. Clearly, they had a special bond as well. And regarding my older brother, he and I have very different personalities, yet Dad was his hero too. Being a doctor, my brother became the go-to guy in the family for medical problems. But for any issue my brother had, he consulted my dad, who often gave him advice that my brother took to heart. Dad showed unwavering support and love to my brother. They had a special relationship as my brother was also my dad's firstborn.

I remember a time when I was younger and we went out to din-ner with Grandpa Joe and Grandma Sadie, my dad's parents. At this time, I had to be ten or eleven, my dad was probably forty or forty-one, and Grandpa Joe was in his 70s. I remember that the table we had been seated at was very close to a wall, and my dad had to squeeze in to get seated. And when he did, there was a nail protruding from the wall, and it caught Dad in the back, causing a bloody scrape. Grandpa Joe got very angry, and I never saw him like this before. He asked for the restaurant manager, and I'll never forget the words he used, "A boy gets hurt, and nobody does anything?" To my grandpa, my dad was still his little boy, although to me he was my dad, a grown man. *Perspectives.*

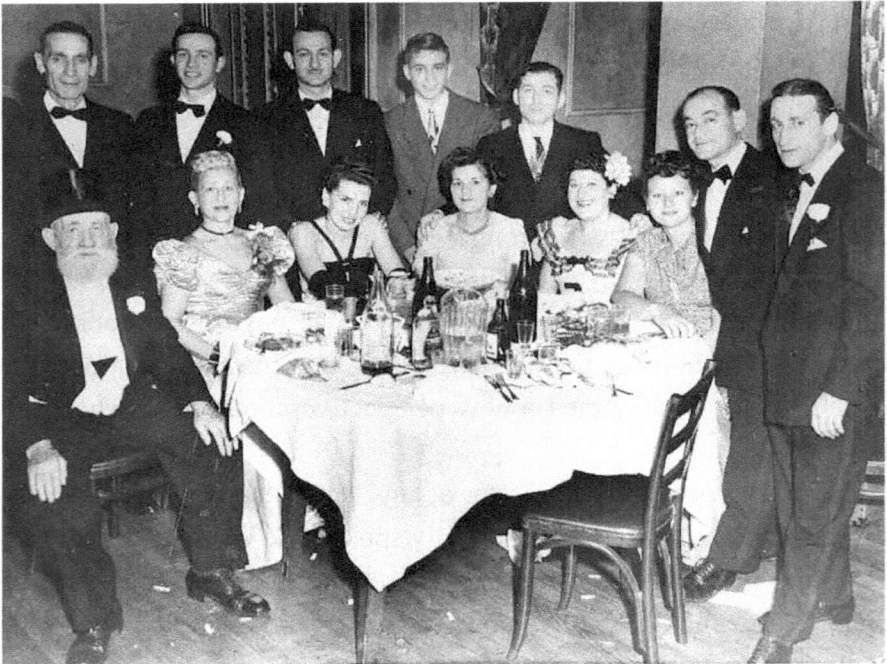

Dad as a young man with his family.

If, as a society, we cannot see another person's or group's perspective, we can get tunnel vision and stay adamant about our own beliefs. If we are fixed on what we believe another person is like, we likely will not be as open to the other's thoughts, ideas, and principles.

Here's an example of this thinking at a sporting event I attended many years ago. It happened on October 2, 1980. That night, my boxing hero, Muhammad Ali, got beaten and battered by Larry Holmes in a heavyweight title fight. It was supposed to be a triumphant night when the Ali of old beat the new "Ali." I went with my best friend and our fathers to see it on closed-circuit TV at Madison Square Graden.

On this particular night, we also had great interest in one of the undercard fights: Saoul "Sweet" Mamby vs. Maurice "Termite" Watkins. We are Jewish and always had great interest in Jewish fighters, especially since there were so few. Although his mother was of Spanish descent, and his father was from Jamaica, Mamby had converted to Judaism at age four. We had never seen either fighter box before, and my friend and I watched the fight with great interest and intent. Before the round fifteen decision was announced, my friend said, "That was a tough fight. It was very close, and Mamby barely won." I replied that I thought Mamby won easily. As it turned out, Mamby won a lopsided decision on all three judges' scorecards. My friend and I did not watch two different fights: we watched two different fighters. We couldn't hear the announcers and he actually thought Termite Watkins was Saoul Mamby. Both of us were so focused on who we thought Mamby was that every punch our man threw looked to us as if it scored points. I started to realize that night that both of us were so predisposed to a Mamby victory that we could not objectively watch the bout.

I didn't plan to get political in this chapter, and my personal beliefs are irrelevant. I submit that there is no such thing as "objectivity" in U.S. politics right now, and neither side can see the other's perspectives. When we accept this premise and find the grey in America's politics instead of the black and white, we can still have meaningful progress in the face of discord.

At some point in our lives, we get predisposed to a certain point of view, or a certain belief or value system. By the time we reach adulthood, this philosophy, ideology, or political allegiance has been imprinted in our brains, and we can only view events through that lens.

In politics, this predisposition manifests itself in partisanship, and both sides can get so "dug in" that the rhetoric can get increasingly loud, intense, bold, and vicious. To make any progress as a society, op-posing sides must find the "grey" that connects our separate black and white. We often look at our "side" through rose-colored glasses, but if we find the "grey," we may be able to accept that opposing points of view may have value and merit. We need to understand and appreciate differing *perspectives* to have meaningful discussions, compromise, and advancement.

Wouldn't it be great if CNN sometimes aired programs from FOX, and FOX sometimes aired programs from CNN? We need to be awakened from our own one-sided view, just like my dad was awakened from his dementia. I would have sworn my dad was long-gone before that day he woke up. His awakening helped me see the "grey" in his medical condition.

In politics or everyday life, being able to understand someone else's point of view, experiences, and beliefs, even a little, will create more harmony in those relationships and can lessen tension when people disagree. Being more open to opposing views and perspectives, and be-ing less entrenched in our own thought processes, could lead us to being more open to compromise and problem-solving. We will also, as a nat-ural consequence, be more empathetic to each other. When my dad was overcome by his dementia, I thought it was all about me, about my loss. When he woke me up, he woke me up to the idea that he was also losing things important to him, among them his relationship with his wife, kids, with me. It's another life lesson I received from my dad that made a huge impact on how I live my life.

REFLECT

Your mind, my mind, can be an open hand or a closed fist. If a person or fate, whatever you want to call it, wants to reach out and hand you a gift, they can put it into an open hand, but not into the fist.

Take this space to reflect on a moment that enabled you to see the grey, that enabled you to be open to a *perspective* different from yours. Or reflect on a time when you were able to help a person open up to your grey, your perspective. When my dad woke up from dementia, he woke me up too, in so many ways. I would love to know that he helped you see a space where you, or someone you love, could wake up too.

Add your reflections here.

Chapter 14

A Living Eulogy for My Father

When I attend a funeral, I am always struck by an odd thought: Isn't it a shame that the person who really should be hearing the eulogy is no longer with us? I have attended my fair share of funerals. I have lost both parents, beloved aunts, uncles, and grandparents. I have been to funerals of friends who lost parents or loved ones. I lost a very close friend. I have listened to many eulogies paying homage to the deceased. I am always moved to tears, whether I knew the departed or not. These eulogies are so heartfelt and touching and clearly express how much the deceased was loved and how many lives they touched. Even when I knew the person, I always learn something new or gain a new perspective or appreciation.

Why is it that most people never *really* express to the people they love or admire how much they mean to them while they are alive? Sure, we often tell each other, "I love you," or say, "You're a good person," or "Thank you for being my friend," but how often do we take the time to write a note or make a speech expressing more of how we feel? Very few of us will receive a "Lifetime Achievement Award" in Hollywood where a room full of people pays tribute to you, but why shouldn't that happen?

I may be an exception. When I turned forty, I became very sentimental and wrote both of my parents a letter expressing how I truly felt about them. Each separately told me it was the greatest gift I could ever have given them. My birthday hugs that year were a little tighter and had a little more meaning. Their reactions to my letters were actually the greatest gift I received for my birthday that year. I got another chance about five years later when I made a speech to family and friends gathered at my father's surprise 75th birthday party. My mother, my siblings, and seven grandchildren all spoke in turn about the special bond they had with my father, Herbie. I'm so glad he got to hear each spoken word because five short months later, he had a stroke that none of us knew was coming.

When my older brother spoke, the first thing he said was that he and my father were so alike. My initial reaction was to think *This is strange, because I am just like my father, and my brother and I are different.* Then my brother explained: he looked very much like my father (check), and had similar traits (check). Growing up, my father was the great problem solver. No matter what the issue, he could solve it. Many times, I would hear my mother say, "Herbie, go take care of it," and, of course, he did. For me, even as I grew into adulthood and middle age, my father played this role. Whether he actually solved the problem or just made me feel better, I felt like he was still solving my problems. As we grew older, my brother picked up the mantle of "day-to-day problem solver," not only for his side of the family, but for his wife's side and his friends as well. Being a doctor didn't hurt, but the ability to make things better came from my father. My brother's speech consisted primarily of three funny stories about my dad.

I spoke next. I said that I, too, was just like my father. I mentioned that I'd inherited his brilliant sales and marketing ability, his confidence, and sense of humor. I focused on my love for him and shared some of the things I had written in my earlier letter. I also said, "My father was the dad who always took my friends to the ball game. I recently ran into a man I hadn't seen in thirty-five years. After recognizing me, the first sentence out of his mouth was, 'How is your father? He was my little league coach, and I loved him.'"

It was then my younger sister's turn. Although she didn't say it, she too is like my father. They both share a love of family and an innate ability to make their family a priority. She talked about how all her friends loved my father. She said, "My dad has the ability to make everyone feel special, so can you imagine being Herbie's baby girl?" My sister sang "To Sir with Love" as part of her speech to Dad.

Five months after this party, my father had his stroke. After his stroke, my father suffered from dementia and steadily declined over more than ten years. I was so thrilled that he'd had the chance to hear his living eulogies from his family and good friends. At the party, my father thanked us all and spoke for a few minutes about his love for his family, but his facial expressions while each person was speaking about him truly told the story.

With the living eulogies, I know that others in his family, and my father's friends who were present, learned many things about my father that they may not have known. Besides hearing some funny stories, they may not have known what a tough guy he could be, how fiercely protective he was of family and friends, or how funny and truly charming he was. Many present gained a new perspective of my dad because their relationships with him were limited to work colleagues, neighbors, distant relatives, or friends.

What do I hope this chapter and book accomplish? If they accomplish nothing more than sharing a little piece of my father with the people who don't know him, that is great. However, if the book motivates you, the reader, to email a note (or even better, write a letter), make an audio recording, or shoot a video about a friend, family member, or loved one, and then *share it* with them, that would be terrific. And it shouldn't be limited to older people. Why not share your feelings, memories, or stories with anyone you feel has touched you in some way? Whether you have known them a long time or met them on a single occasion, and they influenced you, share your feelings. This person doesn't need to be "closer" to the end of their life to hear about how much you appreciate and/or loved them.

So that takes me back to where I started. Why do we need someone to die to share our most heartfelt memories, stories, and love? Why is it often "only in death" that we choose to remember the good and only good about someone? Let s make a vow to share our love and admiration for someone while they are living.

REFLECT

It is perhaps odd to think of a eulogy as something happy, or something for a living person. What it really is may be a reflection on how our friend or family member has truly touched our lives. Not that we need reminding, but often they don't know how much they mean to us.

Take this moment to yourself to reflect on someone you love deeply, and what you would tell them about that if you had no fear of it being a bit strange to do so. Just like writing it here, you can write it in a letter, or email, if it's too much to say it aloud. I loved telling my dad what he meant to me, and I tell my children often. If you're worried, write it here, and we can tell your person together.

Add your reflections here.

Chapter 15
Memories

Dementia/Alzheimer's is a terrible disease that not only robs the individual mentally but physically as well. It is heart-wrenching for the caretakers and family. Yet, today, almost ten years after my dad's passing in 2016, I do not remember the man that suffered, but only the man that lived and thrived.

My dad suffered from dementia as a result of a stroke. This once proud man slowly deteriorated mentally and physically over the eleven years following that stroke. The first few years he had some sense of normalcy. He certainly slowed over that period of time, but could still drive, engage in conversation, play cards, enjoy a good meal, and cherish his family. But, to know dementia is to know what is coming: his dementia progressed to the point where he barely spoke, was housebound, couldn't feed himself, was in diapers, had twenty-four-hour care, and at the end was merely existing. He certainly went through all the stages of this terrible disease. Thankfully, for my family, he always knew who we were.

My brother, the internist/cardiologist, was instrumental in keeping my father alive those eleven years. My dad probably should have died after his stroke, but made a nice recovery. On at least three or four occasions, we went to the hospital thinking he might not survive the night, only to see him make a miraculous turnaround by the next morning. He certainly had a great will to live. Each episode was another blow he had to withstand, yet he continued to fight into the next round. It's no wonder he was an undefeated amateur boxer in the Army.

My brother made sure my father's blood was checked weekly, and if he was dehydrated he got fluids. Kidney failure would not get my father. When he couldn't eat solids, he had pureed foods and liquids, and we were so vigilant that he got what he needed. My brother Ken checked and re-checked his medications weekly, making adjustments with his partner when necessary. At one time, another doctor said to me: "What is your brother doing? That's not your father or the Herbie we all know and love. Don't go to extraordinary measures to keep him alive." Yet despite his condition and that doctor's belief, we wanted him alive as long as we could have him. Toward the end of his life, he would just hold my hand or blow me a kiss. That was enough for me. Those gestures represented the essence of the man he had always been: a loving, caring man. The alternative, losing him even a minute early, was not an option for my family. How many times have you heard someone say, "If I could only have one more moment with my loved one?" We had that with my dad, and we largely have my dear brother to thank for it. In fact, I think I may need to write my brother a letter soon, a living eulogy about what he has meant to me.

The answer as to why I held onto to him so tight is not that complicated. In the chapter called "I Wish I Could Flip a Switch and Wake Up My Father", I urged you to accept and cherish your loved one at all times during the dementia journey. Despite the horrible disease *I knew my father was still in there.* It's hard for me to explain, but as he deteriorated, instead of only seeing his decline, I also saw the strong, vibrant man I loved. He was still my dad. Not a shell of the man he had been, but a man I knew and loved, *still.*

Now that he is gone, the pain is still great (especially on the anniversary of his death), and I still cry often, but as much as I mourn and miss him now, I celebrate him and feel his presence. After he died, my mother could not look at a picture of my father. I had no problem the day after he passed and have none now. I kept two of his voice mails to me where he said he loved me, and although they are terribly sad when I play them, I also get comfort. You see, my father still feels very much alive to me, at least as presence. Not the suffering man, but my best friend, confidant, biggest fan, larger-than-life dad. So maybe, just maybe, my acceptance of my father's disease, my including him in life's activities wherever possible, and my ability to remember and still see the wonderful, vital man my father was even in the throes of significant dementia, has embedded itself in my memory, so I see him this way now, even though he is gone.

I think my awakening from all of this is that part of my ability to handle my dad's dementia and the suffering he and the family experienced throughout this time stemmed from my capacity to hold onto and remember the man he was before dementia reared its ugly head. I think that is a good lesson for me to carry forward when dealing with other types of trauma.

REFLECT

Memories aren't fixed. They don't have to stay a certain way. It's true that our last memories of our loved ones who have dementia, or other mental or physical illnesses, may be of figures reduced to shells of the people we loved, but it doesn't have to be that way. They are your memories, and there is nothing wrong with choosing to focus on the best of them instead of the most traumatic or most recent in time.

Take this moment to yourself to reflect on a memory you're holding onto that does not bring you comfort or joy. Then search your memories for a better one, and give yourself permission to swap it in. Let's save our loved ones with dementia, or other mental or physical illness or disability, from losing all the other things they were, all the other experiences we've had of them. They've already lost enough. What's a great memory you are willing to share with me about your special person?

Add your reflections here.

_____
_____
_____
_____
_____
_____
_____
_____
_____
_____
_____
_____
_____
_____
_____
_____
_____
_____
_____
_____
_____
_____
_____
_____
_____
_____
_____
_____
_____

Chapter 16
Who Is Your One?

In 2020, I was sixty-one years old and had a lot going on. We were in the midst of the Coronavirus pandemic, which had caused me (and probably a lot of you as well) great emotional stress. I had an underlying lung issue and was legitimately scared. I also had work and other issues to deal with. During one of these more stressful times, I said to a very close friend, "I wish I had my dad to talk to." Dad had passed away in 2016.

He responded, "We are our fathers." I knew exactly what he meant. He was saying that we are grown men of a certain age and have gained the knowledge to handle our own problems, and that our fathers gave this to us.

I had another conversation with another dear friend and told her about my discussion with my other friend. She agreed with him and said, "That's right, we have our father and mother within us, and we carry forward the lessons learned from them in our own lives." A slightly different take from my male friend, but a similar sentiment.

After really thinking about what they had to say, I agreed with them, but also disagreed. My dad had been gone for four years at that time, but while living, he was always there for me in every situation that I faced, good or bad. He was *the one* for me. I don't know that I have yet been able to fill the spot my father left when he left the world, or that I'll ever be able to.

Although I may not have completely agreed with my friends, they were right. Through sixty-one years of living, I had experienced the ups and downs of life, and, like my father, was there for my family and had learned to be a problem solver myself. It is true that with age comes wisdom. What that doesn't mean, however, is that there is any statute of limitations on still needing that *one* special person in your life. While we can become a role model for others, that doesn't mean we don't still need someone to guide us and comfort us as well. I'm not sure that my dad could wave a magic wand and make my problems go away, but I do know that just speaking to him would have made me feel better.

As you can tell from this book, I have written a lot about my father. It's not only that I miss him greatly, but he played a role in my life that cannot be duplicated. Hopefully, everyone on this planet has or has had their own Herbie.

Can we define *the one*? If we were to build that person from the ground up, I think we would all agree that this person must love us unconditionally. I believe there are a very few select individuals we each have who love us unconditionally. For most of us, that would include our Mom and Dad. And while my mother loved me unconditionally, and I loved her as much as I loved my dad, she got stressed when I discussed the problems I was going through. My children love me. Your siblings can be your *one*, but they have their own families and issues too. A spouse or significant other can also be *the one*. And sometimes, that role can be filled by a very close friend.

Unconditional love must be the foundation for everyone's *one*. From there, each of us may have different "building blocks" of who and what that person is. When I was going through something (and I have had my share of things, including a divorce), my father would often say, "Don't whip yourself." The message being that no matter how hard a situation is or how painful, recognize that it exists, try to find a solution, but don't let it completely tear you apart. Throughout my life, those words brought me comfort. My dad was my best friend, confidant, and problem solver. He never judged me, but was my greatest supporter.

Does having *the one* in your life mean they are perfect? By no means. No one is perfect. My dad had his flaws and made his mistakes. This actually makes them more human. *The one* in your life knows the things to do and say to you because they know you so well. They never judge you. It's the person in your life who has no ego when it comes to you and wants you to *surpass them.*

When you lose *the one*, there is a void in your life that can never be replaced. I am sure the greatest people of our, or any, generation also had *the one* in their life. George W. Bush, the 43rd President of the United States, called his father, George H. W. Bush, the 41st President of the United States, his hero. George W. Bush often spoke of his respect, love, and admiration for his father, both during his own presidency and in his personal life. How often have we seen professional athletes salute their moms or wave at them when the camera pans to them on the sidelines? I remember seeing the video of Tom Brady, the greatest quarterback of all time, tearing up as he spoke about his hero, his dad, who he looked up to every day.

Hopefully, when you lose *the one*, you have a one-A, or a two waiting in the wings. They might not live up to *the one* in your eyes, but we all need someone, don't we? Or perhaps when you lose your *one*, you are guided by the sentiments of my two close friends who take the lesson learned from their *one* and continue to live a meaningful life by being the *one* for someone else.

In reflecting back on this time in my life, I want to honor *the one* in my life, and this book is part of that journey. I hope that all members of society have someone like that in their life. And the beautiful thing about life is that you can simultaneously have *the one* in your life, while being the one in someone else's life as well.

REFLECT

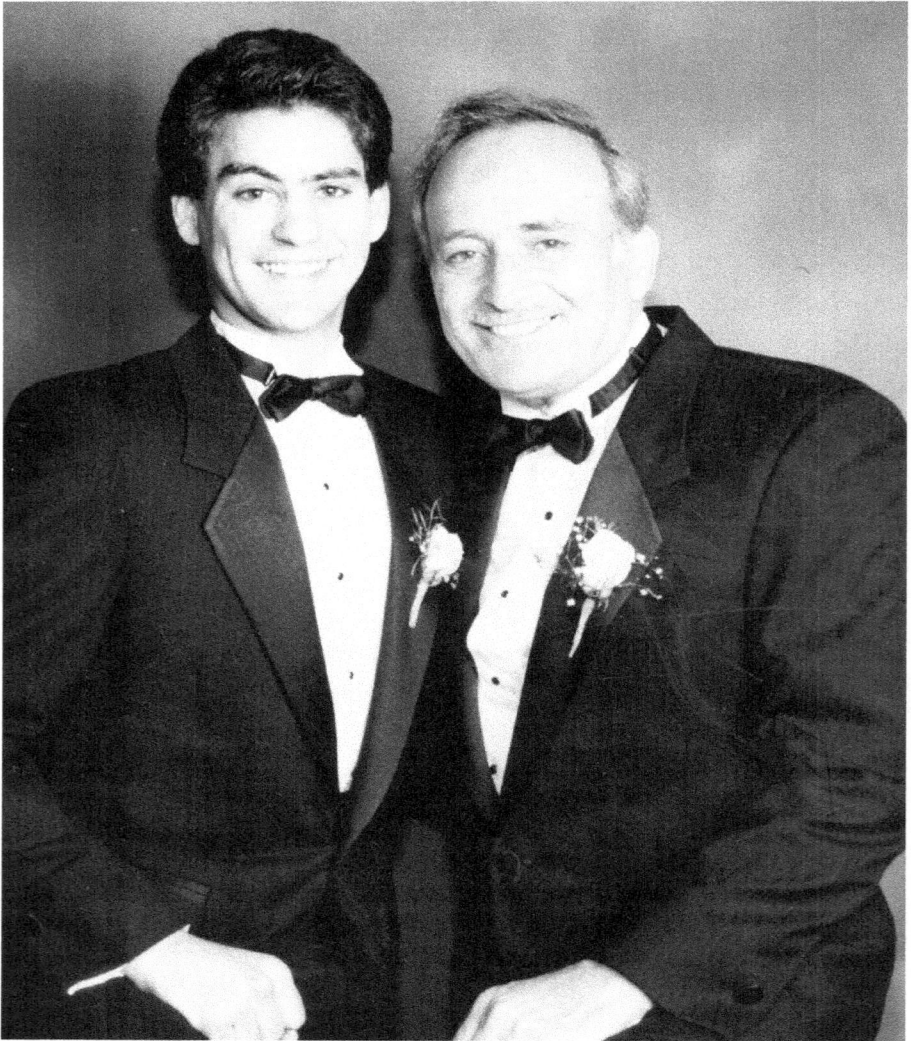

Dan and his One.

Who is your Herbie, and why? Who's the person for whom you're a Herbie?

Add your reflections here.

_____
_____
_____
_____
_____
_____
_____
_____
_____
_____
_____
_____
_____
_____
_____
_____
_____
_____
_____
_____
_____
_____
_____
_____
_____
_____
_____

Afterword

Thank you for reading about my dad, for helping me keep him alive. Thank you also for not giving up on your person with dementia or other mental or physical illness or disability, for the love and care you give every day, for the loss and grief and pain you shoulder, and for the memories you save.

Was there a part of this book you liked the best? I'd love you to let me know. Is there something about your loved one this book helped you remember or cherish? I can't thank you enough for thinking about it and sharing this journey with me.

I hope you enjoyed this book. I'm hoping you take advantage of the REFLECT pages, almost as if you are co-writing the book with me by sharing your own reflections. I'd love for you also to email the ones you want to share with me at info@awakeningsinreallife.com, and I might include it on my website, awakeningsinreallife.com, or as another companion piece to the book and the podcast.

The Awakenings In Real Life podcast features inspiring stories of other individuals' transformation, meaning, and hope. While we typically think of an awakening as a "Getting Up" (Like my Dad's) or as "Spiritual" or "Religious" in nature, an awakening is also an awareness, recognition, or realization of something. We share stories of people triumphing over bullying, addiction, disability, illness, trauma, loss, near-death experiences, and more. The podcast is available on numerous video or audio platforms.

If you have or know of someone who has had an awakening in real life, please reach out to: info@awakeningsinreallife.com.

We are also available on social media.

About the Author

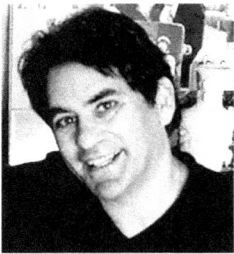

Dan Cohen is a dynamic entrepreneur with over twenty-five years of experience and a deep passion for brand building. Dan is recognized for his strategic approach and ability to foster strong, lasting relationships. With the release of this book, *Awakenings In Real Life*, he tells the story of his dad's awakening from his dementia. When his father awoke, it woke Dan up too.

When Dan talks about "awakenings," he's referring to moments of insight—times of learning, clarity, and personal growth. Exploring his family's past brought all of that forward, and he felt compelled to capture those experiences in this book. His hope is that readers will see parts of their own stories reflected here, enjoy the journey, learn from what his family lived through, and find a sense of connection and meaning. He wants this book to spark your own moments of awakening—or help you recognize the ones already within you—and perhaps even inspire you to share those reflections with the people you love.

Dan is the founder and host of the Awakenings In Real Life podcast. He hopes you will also find it, so you can hear the awakenings that others have shared. They are inspiring stories of transformation, meaning, and hope. Dan is also a speaker and storyteller.

Contact Dan at info@awakeningsinreallife.com

Now That You've Read the Book, Experience the Podcast.

Awakenings in Real Life
New Episodes Drop Every Tuesday

Join me each week for *Awakenings In Real Life,* a unique podcast experience featuring inspired stories of hope, transformation, and meaning. While we typically think of an awakening as a *getting up*, or a *spiritual* or *religious* experience, an awakening is also an awareness, recognition, or realization. My dad's awakening from dementia is the focus of the premier podcast episode and serves as the inspiration for the series. Listen each Tuesday as I interview individuals who have triumphed over different challenges—bullying, addiction, disability, illness, trauma, loss, near death experiences—and more.

**Available on Apple, Spotify, YouTube,
and wherever you listen to podcasts.**

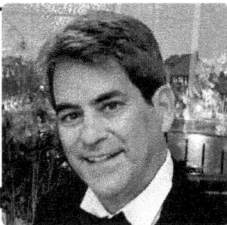

Founder and Host

awakeningsinreallife.com

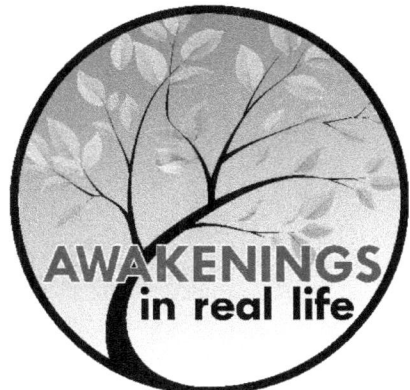

www.ingramcontent.com/pod-product-compliance
Lightning Source LLC
Chambersburg PA
CBHW060230030426

42335CB00014B/1394